LEARNING
TO
SLOW DANCE
With Footprints
of
Kindness

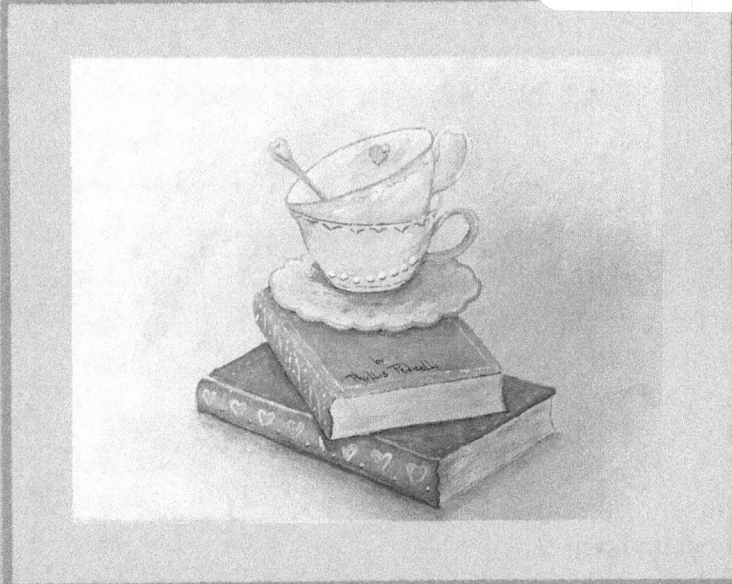

Carol Ann Cole C.M.

Learning to Slow Dance with Footprints of Kindness
© 2024 Carol Ann Cole

Cover art: Phyllis Pedicelli
Cover design: Rebekah Wetmore
Editor: Andrew Wetmore

ISBN: 978-1-998149-39-1
First edition May, 2024

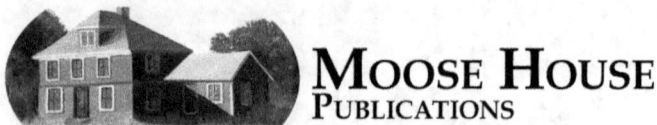

MOOSE HOUSE
PUBLICATIONS

2475 Perotte Road
Annapolis County, NS
B0S 1A0

moosehousepress.com
info@moosehousepress.com

We live and work in Mi'kma'ki, the ancestral and unceded territory of the Mi'kmaw people. This territory is covered by the "Treaties of Peace and Friendship" which Mi'kmaw and Wolastoqiyik (Maliseet) people first signed with the British Crown in 1725. The treaties did not deal with surrender of lands and resources but in fact recognized Mi'kmaq and Wolastoqiyik (Maliseet) title and established the rules for what was to be an ongoing relationship between nations. We are all Treaty people.

Also by Carol Ann Cole

The *Paradise* Series

Paradise
Paradise 548
Paradise on the Morrow*
Paradise d'Entremont Private Investigator*
Around the Corner with Paradise*

Other fiction

Less Than Innocent* (co-author)

Non-fiction

Comfort Heart—a Personal Memoir (with Anjali Kapoor)
Lessons Learned Upside the Head
If I Knew Then What I Know Now
From the Heart (with Deanna Jones)

*from Moose House Publications

This book is dedicated to
My friend and mentor
Mr. Al Peppard
Mr. Middleton
('Pep')

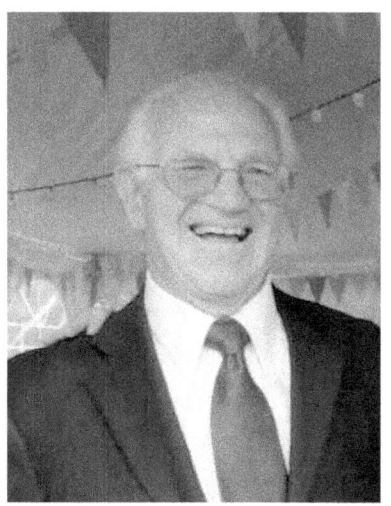

This book shines an enhanced light on past days, throwing some people and events into sharp contrast and prominence which they may not have enjoyed at the time. These are memories shared with a purpose, not court reporting, so there may be some divergence between the events as told and what other participants remember.

Learning to Slow Dance with Footprints of Kindness

Learning to Slow Dance

Introduction

Turning seventy-five years young in 2021 was a big deal for me, for a number of reasons.

When breast cancer knocked on my door the first time, I was forty-five years old. To be honest, I was not at all sure I would live to turn fifty. Cancer came after me a second time sixteen years later. On my sixty-second birthday I was on the operating table once again, and this time I was having the surgery I had been attempting to outrun since my mother's diagnosis and death at the hands of this killer disease.

I am battle-scarred in many ways. I appreciate every day that I have on this earth and I'm grateful for every scar.

In Learning to Slow Dance with Footprints of Kindness I have revisited the lessons I have learned, dating back to my days of growing up in the small community of Wilmot, Nova Scotia. I continue to learn from the Wilmot community and those who grew up with me. I cherish the friendships we formed walking to and from school, playing outside until it was dark and laying the groundwork for lifelong friendships.

I met my best friend, Phyllis White, when she came home from Soldiers Memorial Hospital in Middleton with her mother, Daisy White, just days after she was born. I was three years old when I met Phyllis. Our home was right beside theirs, until it wasn't.

Today, I value the time I spend in Middleton, in what I have dubbed 'my apartment' in the home of Phyllis, and her husband, Tony Pedicelli. Tony has become a good friend as well.

Some of the lessons I learned during my youth and throughout my life have remained firmly intact. Other lessons evolved over time and required updating and an ongoing sense of wanting to 'do better.'

I have always enjoyed having my 'good stuff' in one place…all around me. I have included poems that have inspired me through the years. Additionally you will find quotations that speak to me to this day.

If you're a septuagenarian, meaning you're in your 70s, welcome to my world. We belong to a very special club. No charge to join, just years and years of experience and too many aches and pains to list. I have invited several of my fellow septuagenarians, plus one or two friends who are much younger than 70, to pen brief stories of their own, capturing their life's journey and what life has taught them.

During the Christmas holidays of 2019, like many of you, I heard frightening stories about the 'virus' in China. I remember clearly saying to a friend, "Thank God we don't have this problem here in Canada." I couldn't have been more wrong.

The first quarter of 2020 smacked many of us upside the head and that was only the first wave. I began to spend more time at home, I had my groceries delivered and I reflected on what long-term isolation would look like for me.

And for sixteen months, I did exactly that. I isolated. I remained in my little condo in downtown Toronto, seeing no one. I 'bubbled' with my son and family, who live over an hour away. James called and checked in on me when he could, and he worried about me being so isolated.

This time frame, meaning the pandemic, is when I first began to experience what I call 'a kindness connection.' I received phone calls from individuals from my past, primarily dating back to my Bell Canada days. They were calling to check in and ensure I was safe. I left Bell in 1994, and some of my installation and repair team were the first to call. We had worked together in 1981. Yes, 1981!

This kindness brought with it a yo-yo feeling. On the one hand I felt so isolated, but on the other, I had not received this many phone calls since technology exploded and we stopped calling and began a never-ending discussion online.

Rob Koldenhof called and reminded me of our 1981 days on the same team at Bell. We had such a lovely conversation and I hung up feeling the first wave of this kindness connection. Credit to you, Rob, and thank you. Credit to your wife, Rose, as well.

Within these pages I have left room for you to make your own personal notes and attach pictures if you like. This has been a conscious decision to move over and ask you to join me. There is room for the both of us on many pages that follow.

You might read a quote that reminds you of a personal family memory. Jot your thoughts down here, not on a slip of paper. One day you might want to pass your copy of Learning to Slow Dance on to someone you care about...a grandchild, perhaps.

When you add a few of your own thoughts and memories within the pages, you are indeed part of the fabric of this book.

When you're ready, grab a coffee.

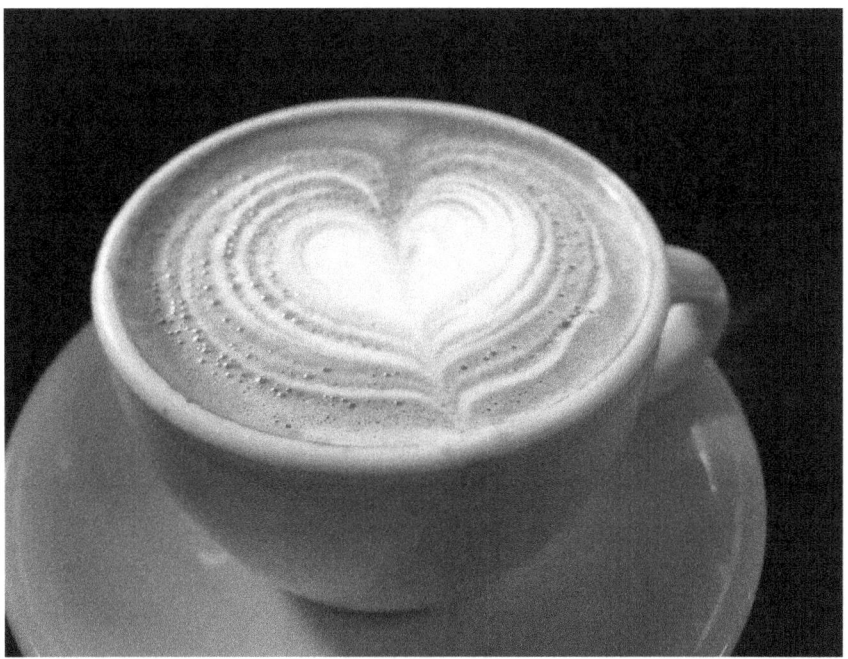

Here we go...

Your thoughts:

Part 1:

Updates to

Lessons Learned Upside the Head

Learning to Slow Dance

1: Soft skills

Years ago, over several careers, soft skills seemed to carry no importance at all. Not even worthy of discussion. I lost track of how many times I heard, "Focus on your measurable performance indicators, Carol Ann, not that soft stuff I hear you talking about." And, one of my favourites, "Sounds to me like soft skills are a women's issue, but I'm only saying that to you young lady."

Today, I am no longer climbing the corporate ladder. In fact, at my age I'm not climbing any ladder. My feet are planted firmly on the ground. (Not counting my colossal fall in 2023. I will get to that later.)

The culture was very different back then. Not a large number of executives, but some, got away with spouting their very personal views. A huge belief of mine was, and still is, that the culture of earlier generations can evolve into a better business model for today. We can learn so much more as we move forward.

Fast forward to today. I know for a fact that soft skills are discussed with job applicants up front. No soft skills…no job offer. It's as simple as that. I hear this from individuals in many walks of life. They understand and they have room for soft skills inside their own toolbox.

An example of one of my own soft skills, and perhaps the one I am most proud of today, relates to names. While in the workforce I consistently made it a priority to learn the names of as many men and women on my team as possible. This was considered a soft skill. Not frowned on, but not rewarded or praised either.

"Carol Ann, the men who work for you do not care what you call them as long as you pay them every second Wednesday." Not true.

It has always been my opinion that if someone approaches you and calls you by name, it's impressive. If you are able to do the same, you make that individual feel important.

Likeability, including calling others by name, is a Soft Skill.
This can often lead to Hard Results.

What is your strongest soft skill? Jot it down here.

Your thoughts:

2: Focus forward and don't look back

I try to not look back unless it's to make a point...a 'one-off', so to speak. Given the attitude that COVID is over, I suggest we look back even less. If you can do it, never look back. As I write this, I am not sure we will ever be 'post' COVID, but there is always hope.

We all have memories we would rather tuck away to be viewed only through the rear view mirror. It's not easy, and beginning in 2020 the world we once knew disappeared forever. We can fight it, but it isn't a fight we can win. The 'good old days' are gone. Forever gone. We (all generations) are the ones who will create new 'good old days', so make sure this is on your list as you move forward. You and I have a clean slate... let's make our words count.

Human nature will separate our world into before and after COVID. It's the 'after' we should be grateful for. We have to reach out and take the hand of tomorrow, and hold on tight.

How will we help erase some of the painful memories our children and grandchildren will have regarding the school days they missed, the feeling of being separated from friends, and the crowded home life with everyone needing a clean space to call their own? Time will help. It's a never-ending list depending on the age and number of children affected.

I observed how my son, James, and my daughter-in-law, Tracey, balanced their careers with a teenage son and a young daughter both learning from home.

My grandson, Jalen, at seventeen, for the most part was okay with completing all of his class work from home. He did have some reservations, given that he and his peers were going to graduate from high school and move on, yet they had been operating, almost 100%, in an online school system. Their in-person communication skills might be lacking as they move forward in life.

It wasn't the same for Lexi, who was not yet a teenager. All of the home schooling and Zoom classes instead of 'in person' work with their teacher soon added up, and many in her class were missing their friends and their teacher. It was affecting their school year. Lexi was not a fan of learning from home and, at ten and eleven years old, she would have liked to go to school every day.

As a member of the Writers' Federation of Nova Scotia I had the opportunity, a number of years ago, to speak with students in high-schools and I was delighted to do so. One teacher advised her students as follows:

> At the end of Miss Cole's presentation, please write a note to her, mentioning at least one skill you have learned from her this morning. Additionally, make an observation about how Miss Cole delivered her presentation to us today. I know a number of you would like to be public speakers so here's your chance to talk with a professional speaker and an author.

Some of the feedback was priceless. Honest and priceless.

"I didn't think you would be so old." For the record, I was in my early 50s. The students were not asked to comment on how I looked, but it seemed important to them.

From a very tiny student, who had sat almost in a shock-like state and literally did not move, came this personal and important admission. He spoke softly as he handed me his note and asked if we could talk for a bit.

"Thank you for telling us that you stuttered as a kid. I stutter so much that I hate to speak up in class. Listening to you speak in front of all of us made me feel like I will get over stuttering too. I pretend I'm just shy, but really I'm not. I might ask my teacher if I could talk to you some more. Would that be okay?"

I assured him I would love to hear from him. I was rewarded with a smile just before he bolted. I suspect he was worried that I might ask him something requiring him to speak further.

I called the school the next day and asked that someone give the young man my business card and encourage him to make the call. I asked that his parents be there when he made the first call since I would like to speak with one of his parents briefly.

He called. We talked. I did speak with his father, and assured him that I was honoured to be able to speak with his son. I made sure his parents had my phone number.

His father asked for some examples of my own experience with stuttering and during that exchange he became quite emotional. Clearly it broke his parental heart that their only child continued to at least try to stop stuttering.

There were other comments about my presentation that were more brief, but interesting.

"How do you remember all that stuff?"

"I think your clothes are very cool."

"I thought you would be younger."

"I bet my teacher didn't think much of your leather jacket. I bet it took balls to wear that and stand up in front of hundreds of students who would rather be outside enjoying the sunshine instead of listening to any speaker. Not just you but I wish my teachers could give us a bit of spare time instead of herding us into the auditorium to fill up every second of our day. And one more thing, I bet my note is way too long. Sorry if it is. Seriously, one more thing, I do tend to get muddied in the past so I like your challenge of moving forward, thinking forward and maybe even being willing to change. My mom doesn't like to change anything and I don't either. Thanks to you and your talk today I am going to work on accepting change."

Finally, and this is one of my favourite comments because it provided what I call a 'teachable moment': "When you asked for my name prior to answering my question, I thought I was in trouble. Now I get it. My name is important. You made me feel proud of my name and myself. Thank you for teaching me that. I'm going to try this trick with some of my friends."

To be honest, I didn't see it as a trick, but I took his comments as a win.

What I try to do when someone I haven't met yet speaks to me, is ask for his or her name before I reply. I do that so I can address them by name at some point during my reply. It's easy to do.

I was fortunate to make a real connection during school visits, with both young women and young men. The connection didn't last beyond a few months, and that's okay. I like to think the students were moving forward and were not looking back.

I mention these quotes from students for two reasons. To make you smile, I hope, and to give you an example of when looking back is a good thing. I keep these comments in my positive memory bank. As the years go by I may not recall these students as often; but when I do, I smile at least as much as I did when I was standing before them, and later when I was reading their notes.

I felt less than successful some time later, when I was asked to speak with a high-school class in Ontario. This class was made up of would-be writers, ages sixteen, seventeen and one or two who might have been eighteen and in their final year.

I understood this was a voluntary class for the students and that they all wanted to discuss publishing with me and hoped to learn from my experiences.

One or two male students proudly carried a chip on their shoulder. They sat with all of the other male students in the back row. Most of the students in the back were already confident they would easily have their book published, have their song in the hands of Tim McGraw, or sing on the next Canadian Idol show.

I did not want to burst their bubble, but I shared how difficult the publishing world can be and offered to give them any number of examples to support this. It was easy to read this class...at least half had little to no interest at all.

Not being a quitter, I went on to suggest that perhaps they should first put their songs in the hands of a Canadian artist. That idea fell flat.

I tried to engage some of the students in the first row and, thank God, they were interested and had their own written questions to ask. I was able to share why a book might be rejected and how they could find out which Canadian publishers might, at the very least, read their manuscript. I gave these young ladies the name of a book that helped me pick out publishers that might be a good fit for me and I invited them to contact me if there wasn't time to hear all of their questions.

One male student behaved like a rude child during my entire presentation. I should have let it go...but I couldn't. I tried to engage him by asking his name and he refused to give it to me. He kept his head down and his fingers on his phone. His teacher was in the classroom so I left that for her to handle after I had left the building!

She observed that I approached him after the class and was dismissed. The student saw me coming and turned and made a fast exit, much to the delight of his male friends who made up the back of the class. For the most part, the boys were all on their cellphones and most of them didn't even look up. They chatted with each other, and not too quietly.

I failed that day with the boys in the back row...and I learned a valuable lesson from the experience. I'll keep most of the details of that lesson between the teacher and myself.

One thing I should have clarified was the teacher's role during my presentation. I assumed she was there to address any rude students, and perhaps an entire row of students on their phones. Clearly, that was not the case.

I have had other opportunities to speak with Ontario students and I have only good things to say about them. I balance the good with the not so good.

It's important to encourage young students to concentrate on moving forward. Think of today, not tomorrow, and certainly not yesterday. Children will take your lead.

Don't look back. You're not going that way.

You can have a bit of fun with this during dinner with your own children or grandchildren. Who can tell a story without looking back?

Learning to Slow Dance

From the Dalai Lama:

There are only
two days in the year when
nothing can be done.
One is called
yesterday
and one is called
tomorrow.
Today is the day
to love,
believe,
do
and mostly to live.

Your thoughts:

3: The art of listening

Respect the quality of quiet

Learning, and relearning how to listen is not an easy task. If we could check and double-check our own listening skills, this would become easier to do. For the most part we are all guilty of this at one time or another. I work on my listening skills every day.

The quieter you become, the more you hear

We often listen simply for a break in the conversation. If someone dares to pause just long enough to catch their breath, we jump in.

See if you can relate to any of the following examples shared with me during a conference in Edmonton, AB.

"Some say I never listen. This is absolutely not true. I do just the opposite. I hear everything."

"Are you even listening to me?" followed by, "Yes I believe I heard every single word you spoke." Often what an individual might hear is background noise only. You have been tuned out.

Hearing is not listening

When someone interrupts rather than choosing to listen to what you are saying, they are telling you that your input is of no value or interest.

Personally, after years of trying to jump back into the conversation after having been interrupted myself, I no longer do that. I don't reintroduce my story, unless they ask, "What were you saying?"

Do you know the letters used in the word listen are the same letters used in the word silent? I remember when I first heard this. I found myself writing both words down to be sure this was true. It is!

Learn to remain silent while you are listening...that's the message. Bite your tongue. Shut up. Stay quiet.

The word 'listen' contains the same letters as the word 'silent.'

I'm still learning to listen without interrupting. I try. Every day I try, and that has to count for something.

Lesson learned. Indeed.

Your thoughts:

4: Dream and believe

She believed she could,
    so…she did.

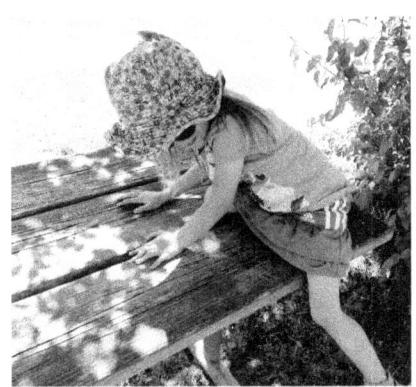

Our children, grandchildren, great-grandchildren are often capable of accomplishing far more than we give them credit for. It's important to keep in mind that they also learn from us.

I have found that sharing a mistake I have made often has more of an impact than sharing a success story. I call these 'teachable moments.'

In the two grainy photos below, Lexi was anxious to show me that she could climb on top of the picnic table 'all by myself.' It was a blistering hot day, with no breeze at all, and I'm sure she made a dozen attempts to get to the top of the table…her glass ceiling for the day.

I repeatedly reminded Lexi that I could help her, but was always met with, "I can do it, Nana. I can do it by myself."

I'm sure you have teachable moments that you could pass on to the next generation in your own family.

Body language in this photo is proof that Lexi could indeed climb to the very top of the picnic table

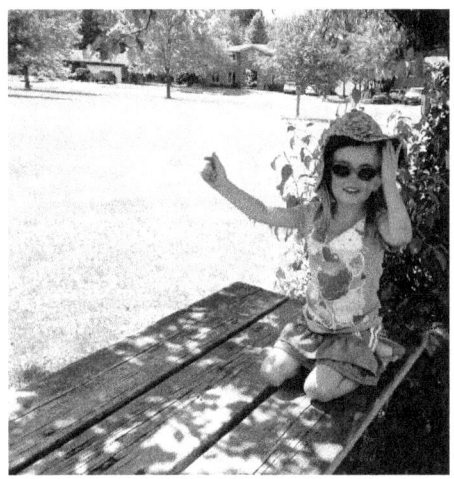

'*all by myself.*' It was a proud moment for a very little girl. "I. Did. It."

Lexi did ask if I could carry her home, and I was happy to oblige. Especially because home was literally just across the street.

I recall during the 80s and 90s thinking, with some degree of pride, that I was opening the door for other women to work and have successful careers, including in non-traditional areas.

I was certain I was breaking the glass ceiling. I was wrong. In fact, I barely made a single crack in it.

We still have not, in my opinion, allowed qualified women the opportunity to hold senior positions in many companies. Women share their frustrations with me. I can relate.

The point I'm making is that I have witnessed the glass ceiling in many companies in corporate Canada still solidly intact. There is work to be done.

Your thoughts:

5: Give the gift of a compliment

The slight touch that comes with a pat on the back speaks volumes. You never know what burden others carry. Not feeling well. Fought with a partner or a child at home. Fought with a peer at work. Financial difficulties. Simply having a bad day.

Don't be greedy in praising others. Show empathy in the work force and at home. Following are a few examples of when you might offer a compliment. It will mean more than you will know.

'Great presentation today. Well done.'
'Nice briefcase. Antique?'
'Good work today. I'm proud of you.'
'Great job cleaning your room, son.'
'Love the new suit. It's very business-like and feminine at the same time.'
'Love the new shoes!' (My favourite.)
'Thanks for cleaning the car.'
'Thanks for the drive today.'
'Thanks for dinner.'

Compliments aren't only important at work. Remember to keep a few for family. Can you add a few examples of your own?

Your thoughts:

From Mandy Haley:

Always show kindness and love for others.
Your words might be filling the empty place in someone's heart.

Nothing is more important than empathy for another human being's suffering. Nothing. Not career, not wealth, not intelligence, certainly not status. We have to feel for one another if we're going to survive with dignity.

– Audrey Hepburn

6: Do not judge others

It's easy to judge someone because of what he or she has said, what their beliefs are, what they contribute, and more. It's far more difficult to take it back once the words of judgment leave our lips.

Often we don't realize we are judging until we speak it aloud. That's almost always too late.

"If he really believes that to be true, then he's the idiot." If you hear words similar to this, remember, these are his/her thoughts, not yours. Don't engage.

"There has to be a reason for all those tattoos." The reasons belong to him/her alone. It's not your body, so stay out of the discussion.

"It has to be his fault. I know it would never be hers." Do you know that, factually? What goes on behind closed doors belongs solely to those who live there. I have lived this mistake. During a casual dinner party, too many years ago to mention, one of our friends announced that she and her husband of some twenty years had broken up. He had already moved out. He had a girlfriend.

As I recall, we all jumped in to dump on the bastard who treated her poorly and left her with all the unpaid bills. Or, so we thought.

> "I never liked anything about the guy."
> "I didn't like the way he treated you."
> "You deserve so much better."
> "Finally, you can now be happy."

Imagine how awkward it was for those of us who had spoken when, a little over a month later and with little fanfare, Buddy moved back in with his wife. I don't know about the others, but I can tell you this was the last time I fell into such a trap. Lesson learned, to say the least.

Becoming and remaining non-judgmental takes concentration, commitment and focus. If we are being honest, we have all judged at one time or another. If, moving forward, we make a conscious effort to not judge others, I believe we will have opportunities to become better people. It's hard work, but worth the effort.

Can you think of a few examples where you found a friend or co-worker to be judging you, or others?

Your thoughts:

Full disclosure: I found it difficult to not judge those who enjoyed protesting COVID health measures a little too much. Whether it's the anti-vaxers, the anti-maskers, the protesters beginning in Ottawa and splintering to other parts of our country...for far too many it soon became their full-time career.

Oh. My. God. They have their reasons. I know they do. I read the papers, I listen to the news and I try my best to separate fact from fiction on both sides. I even follow one or two of the protesters on Facebook, seeking ways I might support them. So far, I'm coming up empty.

> I will not judge.
> I will not judge.
> I will not judge.

At the edge of night, as I recap events in my small world and beyond, it's often very difficult to keep from judging. I still have considerable work to do.

7: Hating only hurts the hater

It took many years for me to understand that *hating really does only hurt the hater*. Understanding this is one thing, but accepting it can be extremely difficult. *Hating is hard work*...I should know.

The relationship I had with my father from a very young age was an angry, hateful one. And for me, it was a heartbreaking one. I'm not ashamed to admit that I hated my father for many years.

When my first book, my memoir, was beginning to come together, I felt the need to be truthful with my father and tell him how honest and raw my description of our relationship would seem to many when my memoir was published. Some who didn't know me well might not believe me.

As it turned out, it was a couple of my own relatives, whom I thought knew me well, who did not support me. I didn't see it coming and therefore had not prepared myself for it.

One of my aunts saw my bruises and asked, "Did my brother do that to your arm?" Yet she chose to tell others I had lied about my relationship with my father when she saw it in writing.

I should have better prepared myself for different reactions to my written words. Don't make my mistake. At the very least I should have prepared my aunt.

The man sitting in front of me the day I decided to share what I had written was blind and in a wheelchair, and he lived in a single room in a nursing home. I had the rough draft of my manuscript with me. I explained what I had written about our relationship and asked if Dad would like me to read it to him.

He said yes, he would like to hear all of it out loud because he didn't recall ever being hard on me. He did go on to say he wasn't interested in the rest of my book, only the pages where he was included.

He was in a very bad mood that day, as he often was when I arrived. He knew I arrived on Sundays and he would wait for me with hate in his eyes.

Dad asked why I had to write about him at all, and I found myself quoting my then-publisher, Jack David, with ECW press in Toronto. Jack helped me understand that a memoir is not a memoir if you eliminate the difficult and painful parts of your life story.

I agreed. My book would tell all, including the tough stuff.

In particular, I shared what I had written regarding the beatings my father inflicted on me from the age of three until I left home at eighteen… for many years with a wire coat hanger and later with his open hand. Always harder than the last time. Always made me cry…initially on the outside, but I learned how to cry on the inside.

Our outside toilet (the old outhouse) was a good place to cry because no one would ever go there with me.

When I finished reading, I looked up at my father with tears in my eyes. I dared to cry openly because of his blindness.

"Are you finished?" he barked at me.

"Yes, I am, Dad. Do you remember?"

"Yes, I sure do remember. I gave you what you deserved and nothing more. I was trying to beat some sense into you. When that didn't work I'd beat you again and I'm not sorry for any of it."

"Okay, then."

I went on to ask Dad if he remembered the summer I took swimming lessons at the old swimming hole near Middleton.

"I damn well do. I remember you failed." It was so like my father to make a comment like that to me.

"Dad, do you remember giving me a hard push back into the swimming hole when you heard I didn't pass?"

"Yes, I do, and I also remember that you damn near drowned. I paid good money for those lessons and it went to waste, because you failed. I pushed you into the water to try again to knock some sense into you. I was teaching you a lesson the only way you seemed to be able to understand."

My father remembered more detail about this than I did, and he said it all with the smirk on his face that I had grown to hate.

It was during moments like this that I truly hated my father more than ever. He had laughed a full belly laugh at my expense. All my years of reliving his beatings and he didn't give me a second thought. Lesson learned.

> ## Keeping baggage from the past
> ## will leave no room for
> ## happiness in the future.

Only when I was able to let go of that hatred for my father could I move forward. I had rented space in my head to this man for decades and decades. I was only hurting myself.

Hating only hurts the hater.

If you have nothing but hate in your heart for a family member, a friend, or anyone else, I encourage you to seek help.

Get professional help, if you are willing to do the hard work that might lead you to the understanding that you are hurting no one but yourself. You might think you have dealt with it and put it behind you. Be sure of that. It took me dozens and dozens of years to learn this lesson.

Finally, choose your words carefully when you make the hard decision to suggest to a dear friend that they might benefit from professional help with the hate they are carrying. They might not see your suggestion in a positive light. I know this to be true because I lost a friend that way. Above all, be sure your friend is interested in your input before you offer it.

Today, mental health does not have to be talked about in a whisper. Nothing needs to be 'swept under the rug.' We have work to do to ensure each and every person takes care of his or her mental, as well as physical, health.

Quote from Gayle King:

> When people don't want the
> Best for You,
> they are not the
> Best For You.

Quote from Drake:

> Haters will broadcast your failure,
> but whisper your success.

8: Honesty matters

A boss once shared that he found me to be *unnervingly* honest. I took it as a win.

A technician shared that he found me to be *brutally* honest. He further said I made him feel uncomfortable.

This same gentleman, I'll call him, 'Buddy', has a wicked sense of humour. During one discussion over more than a couple of beers at a retirement party, Buddy offered an example of how I made him feel. He had an audience of fifteen or more and wanted everyone to know that he had had a meeting with me. His very long single-sentence was amusing.

"Boss, I was talking to the wife about that meeting I had to have with you and I told her you make me nervous because you always say my name like you're reminding me just in case I have forgotten it, plus when you ask me for examples of when you talk brutally honest to me the reason I can't give you any examples is because, like I already said, you make me nervous and I know this all started when I had two 'preventable motor vehicle accidents' over a two-day period but give me a break..."

Buddy went on for another twenty minutes and ended his rant with another rant. This one was about 'the wife.'

"I stopped talking because I wanted to make sure the wife was still with me and, boy, was she ever. All she said was, 'you said all of that?'—whatever that was—'to your boss's boss's boss? I'm anxious to meet her! Are you going to introduce us or should I go and find her office myself? You know I am capable of that.'"

"So now, *that's* got me feeling more nervous than ever before. I don't need the wife saying things to the boss that would likely get me in more trouble. I just know she would agree with the boss before she would agree with me."

Buddy took a deep breath as if he was about to make a grand statement. "Quick...one of you guys buy me a beer...make that two ...I'm parched."

True story.

With very few exceptions, being honest means you're always truthful and sincere.

Be honest.
Be
unnervingly
honest

If you compliment your children, grandchildren and friends in the moment, it will stick. They might be unnervingly honest for a bit longer in their young life. Your grandchild will be proud to learn you are making notes about something he or she said. It's a big deal. Trust me.

When both of my grandchildren were small, and James or Tracey would share with them that Nana was on the phone and would they like to speak with me, the answer was either 'yes' or 'no' and they said both with great honesty and clarity. Jalen in particular would most often respond, 'No. I do not,' and he seemed to say this with pride.

I was somewhat prepared for Lexi's response, given that Jalen had trained me well. Lexi face-timed me one evening and our conversation was brief.

"Hi, sweetheart, what a nice surprise!"

This was met with total silence.

"Lexi, are you there? I don't see you, dear."

"Nana, after you answered I went looking for my mom because I didn't mean to call you and I wanted to ask her if I could just tell you that. It was a mistake. I'm trying to call my friend and I was supposed to call her, not you."

Now that's honesty!

"Should you and I hang up?"

"Yes."

And next came one very long word:

"ThankyouNanaIloveyouNanaIhopeyouaredoinggood-NanaandI'msorryNanaandthankyouforunderstandingNana."

End of....

9: Playing for all the marbles

Imagine any number of scenarios; you're in a corporate boardroom in the midst of making a presentation that could make or break your career; you're on ice playing hockey, third period, last minute of play, winning goal at the end of your stick; you and your family are playing board games at home after supper...at some point you have to make a decision. Are you going to play for all the marbles?

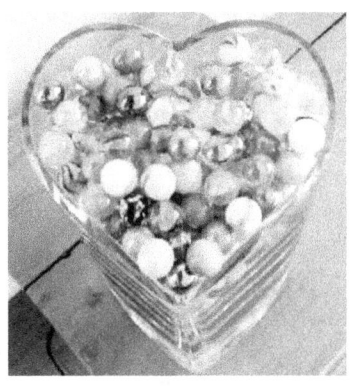

In my case, no matter the job, the boss, or the circumstance I did exactly that.

If something is worth your time and energy, you most likely do the same thing. You might call it something else. "Giving it my all." "Never giving up." "Being all in."

In a lighter look at *playing for all the marbles*, below is my family, doing exactly that on my living room floor.

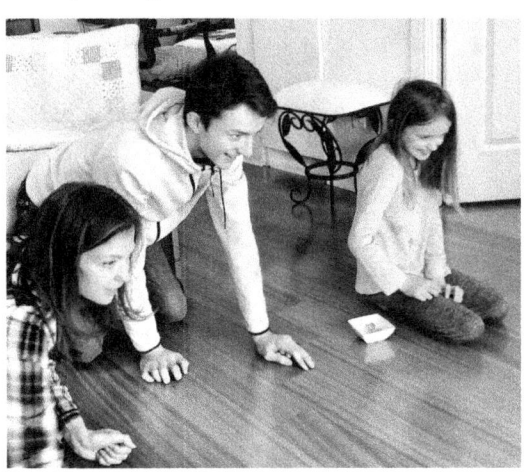

I have a lifelong supply of marbles and a memory to go with each one.

~

I had been in Montreal attending meetings for a couple of days. James was in the city for a few hours, so he dropped in to say hi. He was already playing for all the marbles in his ski career and just getting started.

As James arrived, I was still trying to get home from the airport in Toronto. My boyfriend, Brian, and I were off to a company function and I was already late.

Several days earlier, on the day of my flight *to* Montreal, the cleaning service I used was scheduled to go into my condo and do what cleaning experts do best. At least I knew my condo would be sparkling and bright and the cleaner would be long gone by the time I unlocked the door. My contact with the cleaning service understood that I expected his employee to play for all the marbles.

Somehow there was a huge error in communication.

I walked into my condo to a discussion between three men. *Three men?* My son, my boyfriend *and* my cleaning guy, who almost fainted when he saw me. His eyes were all over the condo while he appeared glued to the floor. Total silence, at least during the first sixty seconds.

Not trusting myself to speak, I turned and walked into my bedroom to drop my overnight bag and briefcase. Having done that I decided to sit quietly and motionless for a minute to ensure I had my anger under control.

One look at my four-poster bed confirmed that someone had slept in my bed. My bed!

I stormed into the living room and first asked James if he had slept in my bed.

"Not guilty," was his answer, so I immediately entered into a heated discussion with my cleaner. It was a brief conversation and somewhat one-sided.

"Get out."

"I'm very sorry."

"Did you sleep in my bed?"

"I didn't think you would mind if I—"

"Get out."

"I really am sorry."

"*Get out!*"

"Can I just wait until my *last load of laundry* is done? Please? I did a few loads of laundry that I brought from home. Again, I didn't think you would mind. You have always been so nice."

"Oh. My. God."

I went to the laundry room, stopped the wash cycle, put it on spin for no more than 30 seconds while I stared straight ahead with a look I would need to wipe from my face before Brian and I left for the party.

Buddy's laundry bag was silently pushed to my feet so I could transfer his very wet clothes, and the washing machine was full to being over-loaded, without slopping too much water on my floors.

Buddy gathered his belongings, which scattered throughout my condo. I was beyond angry. Clearly this young man was not playing for all the marbles or he would have double-checked dates and times and pos-sibly even asked for my return flight number just to cover all the bases.

Mistakes happen. I know that. Buddy should have, at the very least, left his own damn laundry at home until he asked if I minded him bring-ing it along the next time. His actions confirmed there would be no 'next time.'

I opened the door wide and said one more time with feeling, "Get. Out. Of. My. Home."

Leaning on the closed door for a second all I could say was, "Oh. My. God."

I knew James and Brian had stopped talking and were listening to our heated exchange. My son, who, to this day has a wicked sense of humour, didn't disappoint and his timing was perfect.

James looked at me to make sure I was okay, then, speaking directly to Brian, said in a whispered voice that he knew I could hear, "Now you know why I tried to never do anything wrong when I lived with her."

Brian couldn't help himself...he laughed out loud. So did James. So did I.

I still smile when I pull that particular memory from my memory bank. All the marbles indeed...

It doesn't hurt to share how hard we have worked throughout the years. And, if a job was worth time and energy it was worthy of playing for all the marbles.

Do you have a favourite memory that makes you smile? One during which you too played for all the marbles? To be sure you don't forget, write it here while it's fresh in your mind.

Showing our own vulnerability is the right thing to do. I see it as strength, albeit it doesn't always work out. Buddy, my cleaning man, showed his vulnerability when he told me more than he needed to. What really did him in was, "I brought some laundry from home because I didn't think you would mind." No amount of vulnerability would soften my anger with him once those words left his lips.

I do believe in second chances but in this case I needed a bit of time between this man who had slept in my bed and myself.

One of my most vulnerable moments came as I began making a presentation at work. Again, I flew to Montreal to make the presentation one frosty morning, and learned upon entering the corporate boardroom that it might be even frostier inside.

This story dates back to our 'viewgraph machine' days so we're talking old school. *Very old school.* I entered the large conference room quietly and sat at the back until I was introduced or at least welcomed to join the table. While I knew most of the gentlemen present, more than a few were new to me.

My boss introduced me by saying, "Let's take a short washroom break, gentlemen, and then you're up, kid." *That* was my introduction.

I was happy to have the room to myself to collect my thoughts. I wore my newest suit and it was a beauty: sky-blue baggy jacket with huge shoulder pads and big pockets. My suit was 100% silk material and as I deplaned that morning I observed that my suit looked like I had slept in it.

I tried to iron it with my hands as I waited for the meeting to resume. I was aware silk wrinkled easily, but really? There was nothing I could do in the moment.

Matching the colour of my jacket but with an added polka dot pattern throughout the mid-calf flared skirt my confidence was high. I had memorized my presentation so the view-graphs were nothing more than a back-up.

If my presentation went well, for a fleeting moment, I wondered if I could end my presentation by doing a Marilyn Monroe twirl. However there were some powerful men in the room and at least one or two of them would be responsible for my next promotion, so I parked that idea.

I had taken my viewgraphs over to the machine and I double-checked that they were in proper order. I returned to my seat until I heard the men talking outside of the boardroom door. Over the years I would learn that many decisions, important decisions, were made in the men's washroom. *And for the record, I absolutely hate it when that happens.*

Back to my sky-blue suit story. As the men filed back in I stood and lightly brushed my hand over the back of my skirt, from habit more than anything else. My charm bracelet, and don't judge me because everyone had a heavy, noisy charm bracelet back in the day, got caught on something.

I sat back down and tried again. Stand up. Brush the back of your skirt to smooth it. Shouldn't be that difficult, right?

I soon realized my bracelet had somehow got tangled in the thread that ran up and down the centre back seam of my skirt, just below the zipper. God help me! I could bolt or I could show some vulnerability and tell the truth.

Cosmo said, "You're up, kid, and we're running behind, so shorten your presentation."

My one sided discussion went something like this: "Gentlemen, I'm thrilled to have this opportunity to present our BCRIS (a Bell thing) budget actuals for this particular year to-date with projections for the coming two years. I can make this presentation with one hand behind my back, as you can see, or I can fess up and ask you to talk among yourselves while I swing my skirt around so I can detangle my charm-bracelet that seems to have gotten tangled in one of the seams of my skirt."

While the boys were trying to figure out how my comments matched my second viewgraph, I had untangled things in thirty-five seconds or less.

"Okay, we're back in business, gentlemen, and thank you for understanding. I can do this in thirty minutes so you will be caught up time-wise when I am done."

Everything went well and my vulnerability made everyone relax, which helped me relax as well.

My personal confidence took a bit of a beating, but I survived, and I did get the promotion. It took a bit longer than I had hoped, but it did happen.

10: Calls and chances

Growing up with a mother who was always working, always at the office, always trying to climb one more mountain, my son was proud of the fact that he had permission to call my office and have me interrupted anytime he needed me. Anytime!

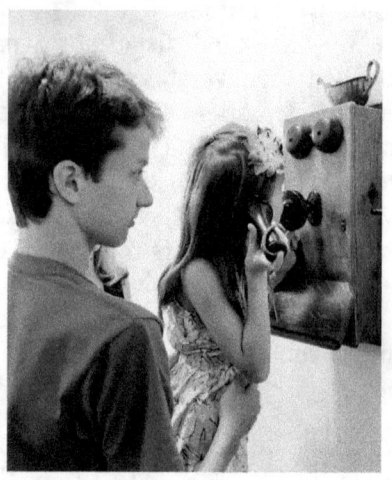

Admittedly, James sometimes called with questions that were not important, but there were many more times that he called with good reason. If it was important to him, it was important to me.

It's a small gift we can give our kids. "Call me anytime if you need me."

Never ignore a call from home.

There are two sides to every story. I know that. During the 70s I worked with a few men who advised their secretaries to check before putting a call through if it was from home. It always rubbed me the wrong way... but one day in particular I learned it was none of my business.

I followed a peer of mine into his office after I heard him saying to his secretary, "I'm in a meeting if 'the wife' calls."

I lead with, "What kind of a marriage do you have if you don't want to talk to your own wife because it might be an inconvenience to you?"

His reply was angry and it was tough to bounce back from. "Your marriage lasted how long, Carol Ann Scott? About five minutes, is what I heard when you first arrived here. I'm not sure that qualifies you as a shrink who offers marital advice."

He then pretended to be looking at something on his desk while saying, "Close the door on your way out."

Ouch.

He wasn't wrong. This was not my business. Another lesson learned.

As I closed the door, per his instructions, I looked over my shoulder and said, "Touché." There wasn't much else I could add.

However, for me personally, I firmly believe, even to this day, that you should always take a call from home.

My mother believed in all good things. In the poem below, she wrote about choices we make, thoughts that we think, tasks that we finish and more....This was one of my mom's favourite poems. I read it to her a few times when she was in the last stages of life.

First I had to find that particular diary, though. Mom had filled the pages in many diaries. In case this is difficult to read, I have repeated the last four lines for you.

> For each of us has a talent or two
> A chance to make good on the job that we do;
> A measure of time to squander or use
> Is given to us...it's our job to choose.

11: Prioritize your time

To this very day, I can't live with any amount of laundry in the basket. I share this bit of information with you in case you think I have mastered everything I have written about. Far from it.

To further illustrate this, when I have an early morning flight (from Toronto to Halifax, for example) I change my bedding the day before, and leave my bedroom looking beautiful from one corner to the other.

So, that last night before my flight, do I sleep in my comfortable bed? Oh no, I sleep on the living room sofa or on the daybed in my den, with one sheet only...half under me and half as my only 'blanket' for the night.

I'm a work in progress and prioritizing is something I have not yet mastered. Remember...don't judge me!

When James and I relocated from Montreal back to Toronto in the mid 80s, I established a rule concerning weekly laundry. Thursday after school/work, whoever arrived home first was to start the laundry. James would tell you, and he wouldn't be wrong, that he would often have all of our laundry done by the time I arrived home from work.

Was that fair of me? No, it wasn't, but James knew how hard I worked so he did what he could at home. Not always without being asked more than once, but he was sixteen, after all. Any time I arrived home late in the evening to find the laundry basket empty, I took it as a win.

In the mid 80s I treated my son and myself to a cleaning lady. And Jeannie was a lady through and through, and so interesting. She is European and there was a time she sang opera in her hometown. What James and I didn't know was that she had a habit of taking her blouse or top off while she sang when nobody else was home, because she liked to spread her arms wide while she was in strong-song mode, wearing only her bra over her large breasts.

It wasn't me who walked in on her. It was James. He couldn't wait to tell me. That was one of those urgent calls from home that I did indeed answer.

Jeannie still comes up in conversation, and always with a smile from both James and me.

This rule isn't really about laundry, as you may have guessed. It's about prioritizing time, all of your time.

Your thoughts:

12: Say you're sorry when you screw up

For the most part, men are better at this than we are, ladies. I've actually lived this. Eventually, I figured it out.

I observed, over and over, during my 'big job at the Bell' days, that men apologize when necessary and quickly move on. They don't repeat the apology because, once they address the issues, they put it out of their mind. Done! They move forward. I applaud them!

I often caught myself apologizing a second time. "Oh I still feel so badly for..." Or, "I have been wanting to talk with you again after our meeting. I hope you realize how serious I was with my apology last week." Blah. Blah. Blah.

Clearly the issue, for which I had apologized more than once, remained unresolved in my own mind.

What I might have been apologizing for isn't relevant. The lesson we need to learn is that there are times, too many times perhaps, when we keep apologizing over and over again every time we see the person we have 'wronged' in some way.

Ladies, we allow ourselves to carry guilt long after we have apologized the first time. I believe we dilute our apology every time we repeat it.

Catch yourself the next time you feel that you should apologize for something. Say you're sorry...once. *Once only*.

When you know it's the right thing to do
Say you're sorry.
Say it once.
Mean it.
Move on.
The End.

13: The face of depression

It's important to never ignore depression. Following COVID and for all the years that follow it will be essential that everyone keep an eye out for that loved one or friend who suffers from depression. Our world is a very different place today, and often a scary one.

Depression is real. When a friend encourages you to forget something they shared with you the night before, I encourage you to be alert. "Oh it's nothing. I shouldn't have even bothered you with it. I'm not really depressed." Keep that conversation going. Don't let it go if you think your friend needs help. Depression is difficult to discuss.

Listen carefully to every word spoken and help where you can. It's not always easy to tell someone that you suffer from depression. If someone comes to you and blurts out, "I don't know how long I can live like this," be careful and considerate in your response. If the particular situation they are facing is above your pay grade, admit it. Then stick with him or her at least until they find help. Asking for help is often the hardest part.

Full disclosure, I have battled depression since 2008. I call my breast cancer surgery on March 28, 2008 my 'strike two.' I discuss my battle with my doctor often and I take medication as required.

Robin Williams left us too soon. He left behind many positive quotes. In many of his quotes I suspect he was speaking of himself and not just about depression in general.

> **People don't fake depression.**
> **They fake being okay.**
> **Remember that.**
> **And, be kind.**

If you've ever been depressed you have probably faked it now and then. Robin Williams also said:

> **Everyone you meet is fighting**
> **a battle you know nothing about.**
> **Be kind.**
> **Always.**

We sometimes have to remind ourselves how little we know about a peer at work or a friend we don't see very often. Life is tough. For those battling any form of mental illness, life is even tougher.

From Simon and Garfunkel...

> **Hello darkness, my old friend,**
> **I've come to talk with you again...**

The above quote is one that a depressed individual might say to his or her mirror image. I have done this more than a few times as I work through my own depression.

For days, if not weeks, following my second breast cancer surgery on my birthday in 2008, I couldn't look at my body, even in the privacy of my own home. One morning, as I removed my bathrobe to step into the tub, I caught a glimpse of my scar that runs from centre chest to deep into my under-arm. I couldn't breathe. I'm not exaggerating when I say I nearly fell to the floor.

The level of depression I felt in that moment was not something I could manage on my own and I knew it. It truly frightened me and I'm glad it did.

It wasn't as if I didn't know the intimate details surrounding my surgery and my scar. That's how depression sneaks up on you. It wears a different face when it enters your world. In my case, it was my scar.

I was not thinking clearly and all I knew in the moment was that I needed help. I called and made an appointment to see a doctor the same day. It had to be that very day.

My own doctor didn't have any available time that day, but his receptionist heard the urgency in my voice and suggested she could refer me to a new doctor who had recently joined the Family Practice at Mount Sinai Hospital.

She is my doctor now and forever.

From James Taylor's *Fire and Rain* album…

> **I've seen fire and I've seen rain.**
> **I've seen sunny days that I thought would never end.**
> **I've seen lonely times when I could not find a friend.**
> **But I always thought I'd see you again.**

These lyrics chronicle Taylor's reaction to the death of his girlfriend in a plane crash.

On a very personal level, have you seen fire and rain? Make a few notes here and you can come back to your own experiences that you might like to share and why. Remember to share even a glimpse of the bad stuff as well as the good. A few words from you might ring true with one of your grandkids, and you will help them without knowing it.

Your thoughts:

14: Can you spare a smile?

We all need humour in our lives. Remember how easily we smiled and laughed as small children, and before we became self-conscious as teenagers, even among friends?

"Never been self-conscious in my entire life." There are times that I don't quite believe that, but if I'm not judging you then I smile and say, "I'm happy for you." If I believe you, I will smile and say, "How do you do it? Honestly, help me understand. Please."

Many of us hit pause on smiling during the early days of COVID because we were frightened. No one made eye contact. No one was in what I will call, "a smiling mood." Wearing a mask dimmed our smiles for a while. In time, we were able to smile again, even from behind the mask.

I smile every time I hear a baby's laughter and I try to keep Jalen and Lexi's laughter in my heart and mind when I'm leaning towards a pity-party. Laughter often wins, if you let it. I have a memory bank full of the changing laughter of my grandchildren.

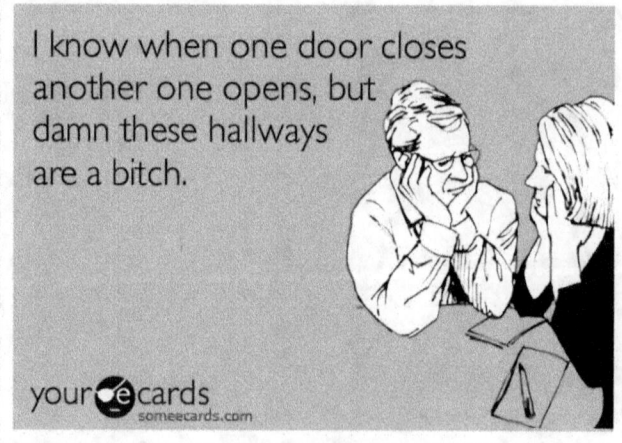

Share your smile with others. It's contagious. Try to laugh often. I have friends I can call and say, "Can you share a smile?" If they can, that's per-fect. If they don't have a smile, that's okay, too. I can easily park my need for a smile while I try to help a friend. Sometimes that's all it takes. Al-ways be honest about how you feel.

Following are a few of the expressions, quotes and musings that have made me laugh more than once over a lifetime. (Sorry about the lan-guage in the bit of comedy on the previous page, Shirley Ambrose! This is the only time I have slipped and said a bad word, I can almost promise you this.)

Be on alert in those hallways!

I think we can also be too positive.

I got called 'pretty' today!
Well, actually the full statement was, 'You're pretty annoying,'
But I try to focus on positive things.

Beginning in the summer of 2021, I have been living in both Halifax and Toronto, and downtown in both cases.

I have friends in both cities who flat-out tell me they are not coming to my home. They simply will not subject themselves to the construction-confusion that seems to appear at every intersection. I understand. There are parking problems everywhere but I do admit it seems I have created my own dilemma by always wanting to live downtown.

Whenever I tell someone where I live and they say,
'OMG, I'm not driving downtown!'
I'm like, 'Calm down. I'm not inviting you over.'

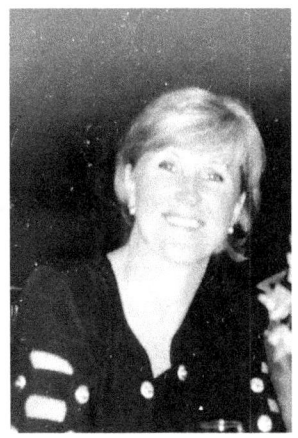

This beautiful lady, Phyllis Pedicelli, is my Wilmot, Nova Scotia, neighbour and best friend. Phyllis has been a part of my life since the day she was born. She is a won-derful artist, and painted the picture for the cover of this book.

I'd walk through fire for my best friend.
Well, not fire, because that's dangerous.
I would walk through a super humid room for Phyllis...
but not too humid
because...well...my hair!

Did your mother use any of the following expressions when you were growing up? I remember my mother using expression #10 on me. It worked. Every time!

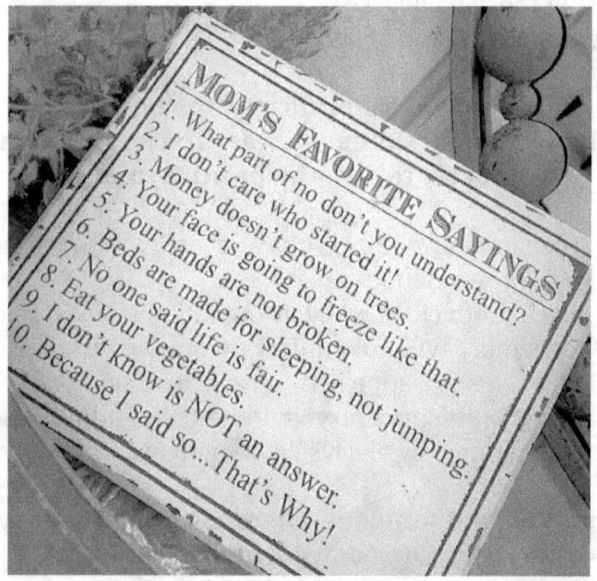

"Because I said so," was often a last resort for mom when I had been re-peatedly asking for something.

"Mom, can I go to Alana's Friday night and stay over? She is having a few girlfriends over to celebrate her birthday."

"No, we have had this discussion before, Carol Ann. You have a per-fectly good bed to sleep in upstairs."

"Everyone else is allowed to go, so why can't I?"

"Didn't you ask the very same question a few months ago? My land, how many birthdays does that girl have?"

"Oh, I was wrong about it that time but it's really her birthday now, I promise."

"The answer is still no."

Turning more negative than I normally would ever dare with my mother I couldn't let it go. "Give me one good reason why I can't go. You haven't given me one good reason."

And then came the closer. "Because I said so, that's why."

Got it!

~

One of my favourite memories involving humour goes back to my early Bell Canada days in North Bay. (With apologies if you have heard me tell this story before...it still makes me smile.)

I was fairly new to the job, and had only recently been trained how to properly ask for payment of an overdue telephone bill while respecting my customer at the same time. We had an answer for everything, and following my training I returned to my desk to begin my 'collections' for the day. I was positive...perhaps too positive and too sure of myself.

The account in front of me showed my customer had a fairly large outstanding balance. I was oozing confidence as I dialed the number. Serious stuff, this service representative job in North Bay in 1965.

Answering machines were fairly new, and when my first call of the day involved listening to a very funny message, an idea was born. I turned to make sure my manager was otherwise occupied. She wasn't at her desk, but that was okay. I decided to live that day to the fullest. The exchange went like this:

"You've reached old MacDonald's farm.
Ei...Ei...O.
Leave your message. I'll call you back.
Ei...Ei...O."

A second time, I looked over my shoulder. The coast was clear.

"I love your funny message sir,
Ei...Ei..O.
I'm Miss Cole from Bell Canada.
Ei...Ei..O.
Pay your bill or I'll pull the plug.
Ei...Ei...O."

Not quite as I had been trained.

We didn't use the expression back then but I'll call what happened next a time out.

First, the door to the monitoring room opened. My manager appeared in front of me. She reached over and hit the button that would ensure I would not be getting the next call coming in to the business office. She pointed to the back room and I followed her there.

We had a long discussion. Mostly, she did the talking. I was to sit quietly and decide if this job was a joke to me, or if I truly wanted to work for Bell Canada and one day build a career for myself.

"You're not a child, Carol Ann, so stop acting like one."

Ouch.

Apparently I had given my manager the impression that this job was a joke to me. As I reflect on this, even today, I can still remember how shocked I was to hear her say that.

I was praying I wasn't going to be fired on the spot. How would I pay my portion of the rent? Even worse, how would I explain any of this to my mother? "Well mom, I had a bit of fun with one of my customers. A customer with an overdue account and..."

Mom would never support my actions. She had already warned me that I had a good job and should keep my head down and do my work with *"None of your silly jokes."* I can hear mom's voice in my head.

When my boss re-entered the room I couldn't wait to plead my case. I loved my job and couldn't imagine losing it over this little bit of fun. Seems we weren't to have fun between 8:30 am and 5 pm.

She stood over me and said nothing. Finally it dawned on me. Her expectation was that I would have something to say for myself.

"Please, give me a break. I now realize we are expected to have *no fun at all* while at the office."

My manager's prolonged silence suggested I must have more to say. Or, I better have more to say.

"I am so sorry. Honest to God. It won't happen again. But, in an era when our newest slogan is, *'Remember to tell, we need girls at the Bell,'* you're not going to fire me over this are you?"

I then followed up with a whimpered, "Ei...Ei...O."

With the threat of having to go to her manager's office (and his office was the only one with four walls and a door!) if I pulled something like this again, I was sent back to my desk.

My Bell peeps laughed about it behind my back, don't you think? I thought it was a harmless bit of creativity. Apparently not!

15: Dress codes

My dress code was simple and it was personal: "Dress as you please and *never* ask the question, 'What should I wear?'"

As I sit comfortably amongst my fellow septuagenarians, I will admit that a number of my purchases back in the day were not meant for the corporate boardroom. One example could be my brilliant red suit. Perhaps it did not need the tassels...one at centre back and one on each sleeve. Additionally, my hemline could have been a bit lower.

I did not *need* to wear leather every other day. Oh, how I loved my leather.

My friend, Mike Bullard, once introduced me at a conference by saying, "Ladies and gentlemen, did you know we have a keynote speaker for you today? This lady is the only person I know who wears more leather than John Wayne...Carol Ann Cole, come on up here."

To be totally honest, I could have lowered the hemline on all of my skirts. And the stories regarding my choice of a bra, or no bra, are best left shelved.

Apologies to my son...

This makes me a good fit as a professional speaker to talk with young ladies and gentlemen today about how they dress and how their chosen outfit for the day might indeed send a message they had not intended to send. I use myself as an example, and this is always a smart thing to do when you are staring into teenaged eyes...laughing at myself makes me a bit more believable as well as relatable.

I encourage you to simply be sure you fully understand what your message of the day is. I will admit there are some who have replied with, "I'm not sending a message to anyone. I'm being me." I try to engage them in a further conversation, but if the interest isn't there, I move on. After all, I've been there.

I recall the embarrassment I felt when I was visiting another Bell office in the late 70s. I was presented with a jacket because, "Carol Ann, your arms are showing. I will ask you to wear this jacket while you're with us. We have an office dress code and sleeveless is not permitted." I opted to cut my day short and leave rather than wear their coat of shame one minute longer than necessary.

Looking back, do I have any regrets regarding my style? Not a one. It really was a different time, though.

Somewhere along the way between then and now, it seems entertainers, Beyoncé for example, rewrote the book on proper attire for young women. The basic piece of clothing is a second-skin bodysuit that has high-cut legs and low-cut chest, and to each his or her own to accessorize with tassels or glitter or nothing at all. The only rule seems to be "Keep your crotch and nipples covered" for females and "No bare crotch" for men. (I know...my age is showing!)

Dress as you please.
And always, always, understand the message that you send.

Do you have dress-code memories of your own? Jot your thoughts down here, not your thoughts about how I dressed but memories of how you dressed or perhaps a discussion you were part of back in the day.

Your thoughts:

16: Be nice

Everyone deserves a second chance.

I try to keep this in the back of my mind, ready to pull it from my memory bank at a moment's notice.

We have all heard the rants from friends and co-workers: 'That's it for me, I'm never going to believe a word that comes out of her mouth.' Or, 'That's the very last time I will offer to help him.' Finally, 'Whoever said that being nice to everyone is a *good thing*?'

Over a drink with a friend some fifty years ago, I asked how many 'last chances' he figured he had been given during his career. Wearing all of his last chances like a badge of honour, he proudly ran through a dozen or so. However, when I asked how often he had given others a second chance, he had difficulty recalling even one time.

It works both ways.

If you're unsure, give the benefit of the doubt and be nice a second time. You might be surprised at the result.

I admit there are times when you can be nice twice, three, four and five times and it still doesn't seem to make a difference. Don't count this person out until you are absolutely sure they don't deserve your support one more time. Additionally, you decide how many chances you can spare and give only the number you feel are deserved.

It goes back to not knowing what someone may have faced at home prior to walking into the office, greeting no one and sitting at their desk staring into their coffee cup. This peer's mood most likely had absolutely nothing to do with you or with their workload. You can't 'fix' everything for everyone, but you can always decide to give out one more chance.

How do you handle conflict within the walls of your home? I hope you give family members a second chance. I realize second chances within some families just won't happen for reasons that we don't and can't understand. The quiet pat on the shoulder at day's end is a place to start while you look for commonality. "It's been a long day, son. Time you were in bed, don't you think?"

One word of caution...never let anyone take advantage of your generous heart. I have allowed that to happen in my world, and that's on me.

All I ask is that you...

Be nice.
Twice.

Your thoughts

17: The first cut is the deepest

I began writing this story in 1966. Until now, I have not shared this level of detail. Other than writing all of this in a very personal journal I called GBS, I have been able to compartmentalize all of it...I learned how to do that from my mother.

My journal at the time was a Bell notepad. A form '188', I believe. Secrets for my eyes and ears only...until now.

I was certain I knew what I was doing. I was twenty years old, after all. No longer a teenager. No longer making bad choices. My mindset at my young age was, 'I'm right and everyone else is wrong.'

Graydon Brian Scott and I met in the summer of 1966 on a beach in North Bay, Ontario. We looked great together...something that seemed to be important to both of us. I was twenty and he was a few years older. We married the following year, August 5th, 1967 and our son, James Brian Scott, was born on New Year's Day, 1969.

Simply put, Graydon and I were two strong-willed personalities caught up in a young and immature relationship. This was my first. Graydon was my first. For Graydon...not so much.

By the end of 1969 Graydon and I were barely speaking. We talked through our son. "Maybe mommy and daddy should take you to the beach today, Jamie. How does that sound?" Or, "Jamie, how would you like to taste your first ice-cream? Mommy will get you ready to go and she can come with us if she wants to."

We were living under the same roof, but we were not living together.

Early in 1970, on a cold and frosty Sunday morning, Graydon was packing his hockey gear for a game later that day. Jamie was playing and entertaining himself.

"Tell Daddy we are off to get you into warm clothes before we go to his hockey game."

Graydon followed us into Jamie's room. "I don't want you bringing Jamie to my sports games, starting with hockey today."

I stared at Graydon. Was it possible he had the guts to say what we both knew was happening?

"I'm not comfortable having Jamie at the rink and always yelling, 'Go Daddy'."

"I don't think I understand what you're telling me, Graydon." I realized what was coming. I was just stalling for time.

"Carol Ann, you know I can 'chirp' with the best of them and a lot of that goes on at all sports games. So, I don't want him there."

"Really?" was all I could say.

"Sorry, but—"

I realized Graydon wanted both his wife and his son to disappear. "Don't you dare start with 'sorry', because we both know you're not sorry or you wouldn't be embarrassed to have us cheer you on. I'm guessing it's hockey, baseball, football, etc. Did I miss anything?"

"We've talked about this," Graydon said. He wasn't wrong, but our idea of communication was both shallow and juvenile.

I remained silent.

Graydon continued, "You're not happy. I'm not happy. Thankfully, Jamie is happy enough for both of us. I'm not saying I want you 'gone', but I've moved on. Carol Ann, I made a mistake...a mistake that you refuse to forgive and forget. *One mistake. One lousy mistake and I'm sorry*."

"At the risk of repeating myself, Graydon, you broke our marriage vows, and you're right, I can't forgive you and I can't forget. I have tried. It's not that I won't but that I *can't*."

I was crying and so was my husband.

"You got caught, Graydon, and that's why we are at this point today. You did this."

Graydon was right. I had been thinking about this for several months. I was truly unhappy. Had we made even a cursory attempt to save our marriage? We had not.

Graydon had an affair. There were other affairs that we both pretended I knew nothing about. I simply could not speak the words. He knew that I knew.

I offered a solution and Graydon was relieved. I could see it in his face. "Tomorrow I'll be at work and Jamie will be at day care. With your shift work I know you are off tomorrow, and maybe Tuesday as well? When we arrive home tomorrow, I want you gone. If you are still here, Jamie and I will find a place of our own and we will move out. However, with our son knowing only this place as his home, I believe I should stay here with him, so I'm asking you to move out. *Tomorrow*."

"I'll move out in the morning. It won't take me long. I would like to pick Jamie up early so I can spend a bit of time with him and then we will pick you up after work. I'll just drop you both off."

Father and son picked me up and the silence was deafening. No one spoke a word. Not even young Jamie.

I was grateful as Jamie and I entered our little apartment and looked around. True to his word, Graydon took his clothes and anything in the apartment that he wanted or would need. There was nothing missing that Jamie would notice, so I knew I had time to explain what was going on.

Jamie and I were free to make it *our* apartment and we did exactly that. *All night long.* We had a party that Monday evening and it went on for hours. It was a private party for two: me and the boy.

Our dinner menu was perfect. This was a celebration. Kraft dinner, potato chips, chocolate, and apple sauce...lots of applesauce. Add a side order of toast for two. To drink we proudly ordered (we were pretending we were in a restaurant) Pepsi for mommy and milk for Jamie. My son didn't know what we were celebrating but that didn't matter. There would be time for explaining.

I had a surprise treat for Jamie when we were a few hours into our late-night job. We had jellybeans! Five for mommy and five for Jamie. And many more for mommy once Jamie was sleeping.

Our party involved eating while we worked, which was a novel idea for Jamie. We were not at the kitchen table, so clearly this was a celebration.

I decided we would rearrange the living room furniture, and Jamie's job was to help me decide where everything should go. I wanted him to get up in the morning and feel proud when he came out of his bedroom and walked through our living room.

We made decisions together and we pushed and pulled each piece of furniture back and forth. There was not much room to change anything, to be honest, but we tried. We had the music on and we danced like there was no tomorrow.

Jamie made my heart sing!

By the time we were finished we had moved every single piece of our living room furniture...all part of a 'Bad Boy three-room-grouping' that Graydon and I had picked out as a couple. There would be no tomorrow for this family of three. It was official: the two of us, Jamie and mommy, against the world. Surprisingly enough, I was 100% confident we could do this.

We weren't going to change anything in our bedrooms, so that left the kitchen to work on. I declared the kitchen was for another day.

I had made a decision somewhere during the night that both Jamie and I would stay home for *one* day. I knew my manager would understand. I asked her to not share my news with anyone other than her boss.

My separation from Graydon would make for great gossip and I wasn't looking forward to that part of my immediate future. I was about to hear stories from all four corners of North Bay because 'Scotty,' as Graydon was known, was a beloved athlete who could do no wrong.

Not one, not two, but three hearts were broken. Possibly others, too…

That first cut was deep, lasting, heartbreaking and, yes, life-altering.

One of Graydon's friends in the military, Art Cardinal, had a second job as a singer for a local band. I didn't know this when a few close friends suggested they would like to take me out for a drink or two, because they were worried that I wasn't smiling much. As luck would have it, we selected the very motel where Art was singing. I wasn't overly concerned because many months had passed and I too was entitled to go out.

As soon as he saw me he stopped the band. I knew what was coming… whenever Graydon and I were out and Art was singing a few songs, he would proudly sing, 'Sweet Caroline' with the words changed to, 'Sweet Carol Ann.' I always found it to be a sweet gesture.

Art disappeared when the band took a break, and when he reappeared he headed for our table. I didn't have a chance to say anything about Art to my friends. It wouldn't have made any difference in the end.

"Carol Ann, I have done a stupid thing. I just called Scotty and told him you were here. He was furious and asked me to make sure you didn't leave. I am telling you this because I disagree with Scotty. I think you should get out of here as soon as you can. I'll lose my job with the band if Scotty makes a scene, and he will if you are here."

My friends and I got up and left without a word. I was disappointed in Art that day, but my discussion with him would happen another time.

During the summer of '73 Jamie and I were able to get out of town. Bell transferred us to Kingston, Ontario. My new job came with a promotion, so it was all good!

And the most exciting news of all was that my sister Lois and her husband, Allan Young, along with their young daughters, Natalie and Dawn Marie, were also transferred. They would be moving from Comox, BC to Kingston.

To have the opportunity to live physically closer to one of my three sisters was an incredible gift, especially at that particular time in my life.

I felt very alone and had not yet learned to enjoy my own company. I knew I had to square my broad shoulders and take it on...all of it ...but I had to start with baby steps.

Lois was an incredible help to me when I had to travel to Toronto for meetings. Jamie would stay overnight with his cousins and he loved it. In return, Natalie and Dawn Marie would stay with us during weekends as often as we could manage. Yes, even as far back as 1973 children had busy weekends.

Dawn Marie had, and still has, the most beautiful curly hair. She kept asking me to comb it straight. "My mother combs it straight." She would not back down and was getting a bit loud so we called her mom.

Problem solved: "Just turn her away from the mirror, comb her hair for another few minutes and tell her it's straight. Just don't let her look in the mirror."

Worked like magic. Mother does indeed know best.

Your thoughts:

18: Singles or doubles?

I have always been annoyed when I hear someone whisper the term 'single parent' in a condescending way. It's the whispering that makes it sound as if a single parent is to be pitied.

"I know her son acts out, but what you may not know is that she is on her own. She's a single parent, and at such a young age. I wonder what went on with those two? So many people around here love Scotty. How will she ever make ends meet?"

While having pizza at Valenti's restaurant in North Bay with Jamie and our weekend guests Gaye and her young daughter Dayna Scott, I overheard comments coming from the booth directly behind us. I recognized the voice of my friend Ruth.

"From what I hear, and don't quote me, but Scotty isn't going back to her. I know for a fact he quickly moved in with a student at the college. Sadly, I'm pretty sure Carol Ann is holding out hope that he will, one sunny day, walk back into her life, just like that. That's not going to happen."

While I was listening, I wondered if perhaps Ruth had hoped I would hear her. I had thought until this moment that Ruth was a friend of mine. I assumed I was wrong, but when I gave it more thought I, much later, decided that maybe Ruth couldn't find the words or the courage to face me, so she chose an alternative way to share. I gave her credit for the smack upside the head when we spoke some time later.

Back to that evening at Valenti's restaurant...while I was eavesdropping, Gaye was trying to keep Dayna and Jamie quiet and focused on their supper. She had only heard parts of the whisper. I filled her in once we got home.

Gaye and I were married and separated around the same time. Gaye is Graydon's sister. By the time we were on our own, or 'single parents', as many called us, Gaye and I had become friends and to this day we have remained close. Gaye is more a sister than a sister-in-law. Sisters are forever. I appreciate her so much.

Bell transferred me to Kingston in 1973 and on to Ottawa in 1975. Jamie and I were enrolling him for school that September. Upon learning I was a single parent (her words not mine) the Sister handling enrolment said, "You are Catholic, correct?"

Jamie answered for me, and I couldn't have said it better myself. All in one word he said, "We'reCatholicbutwedon'tgotochurch."

Perhaps you have a single parent in your own family who can relate to my rant?

There are many parents who have had great successes in their lives and so have the 'poor young children' of intelligent women and men who did it on their own...parent and child, hand in hand, taking on the world.

We don't use the term 'two parents' so, in the name of the Lord, could we drop the *single parent* term? *Please*...

Your thoughts:

19: Every story has two sides

When I revisit memories of my time with Graydon, and how excited we were to get married and set up our tiny apartment after our wedding and the wonderful feeling that came with the birth of our baby boy two years later, it's hard to admit how epic our failure was. I still think we had potential. We just didn't know it at the time.

Through the years, I wondered if Graydon wanted to hear stories about Jamie as he began his schooling. I decided on my own that he didn't care about us. That was wrong of me, and I admitted my mistake when speaking with Graydon decades later. I did suggest that the phone lines work both ways. He didn't disagree.

Graydon eventually settled down and married a wonderful woman. Like Graydon, Christine had been married before. She brought three young boys to her second marriage. Paul and Michael were a bit older than Jamie and Sean. Sean and Jamie are the same age, with only months between their birthdays.

Jamie started going to his dad's more often. He would return home so happy and he marvelled that each time he went to visit it seemed like a party with *four* boys in the house. Oh My God, I could not imagine that!

Over time, I learned how much Christine loved her ceramics classes. One year after spending New Year's and his birthday with Graydon, Christine and the boys, Jamie arrived home with a gift for me. He mentioned more than once, as I was opening the gift, that it was from him. It was a beautiful ceramic Christmas tree with all the beautiful lights.

As I finished opening it, Jamie said, "Well, I guess it's really from Christine, right, mom?"

I tried without much success to convince him that Christine made this beautiful tree and she gave it to him and he gave it to me, so it was a Christmas gift from him. He never did buy that logic.

When any marriage breaks down, I think some of the questions our small children put to us tug on our heartstrings. At the end of summer vacation one year, when Jamie came home from his dad's it seemed he had something to tell me. We were just finishing supper when I asked Jamie why he seemed to be looking at me almost with pity on his face.

First I had to explain what 'pity' is.

Then he asked his question, "Mommy, did you know my dad is going to marry Christine?"

Fortunately, I was prepared. "I did know, son, but why does that make you sad?"

His next question was so innocent, and I can still see the look of pity as he finally shared what he had brought home in his heart. "Why doesn't Dad marry you?"

I believe I replied with what any sane mother would say: "That question is best answered en route to Dairy Queen. Put your dishes in the sink and let's go!"

As the years passed, Jamie became James and he continued to spend quality time with his dad, Christine, Paul, Michael and Sean. I don't recall James ever using the term 'half-brothers.' Suddenly he had three brothers, and that made him both proud and happy.

Sean came to visit us in Toronto, and I believe he came to Montreal once as well. Sean was smart and a very kind young man. He had perfect manners and a smile that would melt your heart.

It's not my story to tell, so I will only say that cancer took Sean away from his band of brothers at a young age.

Sean's immediate family and his brothers and their families do a good job of keeping his memory alive. They always will. I'm very proud of the four brothers and I will always include Sean in the mix. When someone passes away they are forever still part of the family.

When my career took James and me to Montreal for a couple of years, I once overheard James conversing with a friend of mine, David, who came to pick me up. David was taking me to dinner. They were downstairs circling each other, so to speak. James was thirteen and very protective of his mother. He still is.

"So, James, it's really great to meet you. Your mother speaks about you often...*a lot, actually.*"

His attempt to crack a joke fell flat. James said nothing at all.

"Do you have any brothers or sisters, James? I believe your mom told me there are just the two of you. Did I get that right?"

"No!"

"No, what?"

"No, you did not get that right. I have three brothers. You must have forgotten that part of the discussion with my mom."

"I would never forget that part of a discussion with any woman, James. Your mother definitely told me you were her only child."

"I am."

I had heard enough from the two children downstairs. "Play nice, boys. I'll be down in a minute."

"Just ask my mother. She'll clear it up." James loved this. "I'm not wrong. Just answering your questions. Sean is my age, Michael is older and Paul is even older than that."

"Okay, I'll ask your mom. Count on it. I don't like being lied to."

"Do *not* call my mother a liar." James stopped the argument because he knew he was winning, and that was enough.

I came downstairs with a smile for James, so he knew what was about to happen. "Son, does this ever get old for you? You have had way too much fun with this today. An apology might be in order, don't you think?"

"Sorry, buddy...but this is going to be much worse for you."

"Son, I am going to walk David out, I'll be back in a second."

I leaned in to James' ear to add, "Don't pull your, 'I told ya' line out or, trust me, this will not be funny."

Slipping his arm around my waist, David said, "We can talk about this over dinner."

However, he clearly could not wait another second. "Four sons? Four? Honestly, you forgot to mention that? What is going on with you, Carol Ann?"

"What part of interrogating my thirteen-year-old son did you think was okay?"

I went on to explain the history of the four brothers. Finally, it seemed totally clear and all was forgiven. Or so he thought.

I said some things that I won't bother to share. It was not my finest hour, but David left knowing that in fact James does have three brothers, and on occasion Sean has visited with us, and that they are all fine young men.

David left without having acknowledged that quizzing the teenaged son of the woman you are picking up to take dinner is not a smart thing to do.

I did run into David at a bar in Montreal a short time later. He didn't see me initially, so I had a drink sent over to him with a note that read, "Dated any young ladies with four sons lately?"

We had a drink together and all was forgiven. Life is too short to sweat the small stuff.

70

20: Fool me once...

I'm ashamed to say that I learned more about Graydon at his funeral than I knew about him on our wedding day or throughout our brief and troubled marriage. We should have known better. *Both of us.*

Graydon and I had discussed *nothing* about my job or his job as an Air Force Policeman (AFP, for those military types reading this). He didn't have any idea that I had a goal to be part of the management team with Bell one day, and that's on me. I didn't mention any of my goals until it was too little too late.

We talked about sports. Nothing else. Graydon was a gifted athlete. He could play any sport better than most. I'm embarrassed to say I was so proud of my husband, yet I really knew nothing about him. I would brag about him at every opportunity, but other than sports...I had nothin'. Sharing this is not an easy thing for me to do and this chapter, among others, is difficult to write.

Graydon lived on the Air Force base in North Bay and I lived downtown at 409 Main Street West with my dear friend, Shirley Ambrose. Graydon and I married within a year of meeting. His boss, Herb Foss, made sure we had the date we needed booked at the Junior Ranks Mess. He and his family had loved Graydon, beginning with their time together with the Armed Forces in Germany. He could do no wrong in their eyes. Their son, Jeff, was Graydon's 'bat boy' at the baseball diamond and Graydon was his hero.

Close friends warned me against this marriage up to and including my wedding day. My Uncle, Seldon Cole, picked me up #409, as Shirley and I called our place, to drive me to the church on time. Uncle Seldon surprised me by saying if I wanted to keep driving he would tell me more about why my marriage should not happen...at least not so soon after meeting each other.

I was beyond upset that my uncle would treat me this way on my wedding day. I said I would listen for a few minutes and I did. Ultimately I refused to accept anything Uncle Seldon was saying. Everyone was just jealous...oh, how young I was. Those who had told my Uncle all these fake stories were just jealous of what we had. I know I made my Uncle feel badly with my wedding day rant. I said someone was lying and I hoped it wasn't him.

He finally said, "Okay, kid. We are off to the church."

Several months into our marriage, I still wanted to have a career rather than a job. I had forgotten to discuss this or any of my goals with Graydon. And if he had any goals for his future, I didn't know what they were. Again, we didn't communicate.

I thank my mother, who always listened when I talked about what I wanted to do with my life. When I mentioned a specific job, she always asked me the same question: "Is that a career or a job?"

A few short months after Jamie was born, I had to admit to myself that Graydon and I were not going to make it as a married couple. I regretted having told my manager at Bell that I was quitting my job. I remember telling Carolyn Passmore that I would not be returning to work after my baby was born. I planned to put all of my focus on being, 'Wife and Mother of the Year.' And I said it with such pride.

In retrospect, I'm embarrassed for my younger self.

I was truly in love with Graydon. I was confident that once our baby was born and I was used to the big change of not only being a mother, but a stay-at-home wife, we would make time to talk about our hopes and dreams.

I grew up considerably following Jamie's birth in 1969.We were in the hospital for an extended period of time and, as busy as the hospital was, I had lots of time to think about my future. About our future.

I remember the day we were discharged from the hospital. We drove home, a family of three, in total silence. After only seventeen months of marriage, I realized Graydon's love for me wasn't a priority for him. I had been kidding myself to think otherwise.

The first time I heard a rumour concerning my husband, who had been out with the boys the previous evening, I was incensed. I told my 'friend' that she didn't know what she was talking about and that one of our other friends was a liar. I apologized to her some years later.

Women gossiping about women is a double-edged sword. One day you gossip and the next day you're the person being gossiped about.

~

My failed marriage left me vulnerable as it related to meeting and trusting other men. I have not spoken of this and certainly never put it on paper. If I didn't have the emotional tools to realize that my husband didn't love me the same way I loved him, then how could I ever fall in love again? It seemed that I didn't know what 'in love' was (not that I'm quoting King Charles).

Given how epically our marriage failed, how would I know if and when 'the one' came along? I didn't trust my own judgment.

On the nights that I let my mind wander to life alone and what that would look like when I retired from Bell, Ruth Bilbia's words rang true, "Carol Ann, I hear you are working both day and night and I'm worried about what you are doing with your life. Bell's BOP [Business Office Practice] will make a very cold bed partner as you move on and move up in your career." I didn't believe Ruth at the time. Today it's easy to admit that she wasn't wrong.

I did meet some wonderful men over the years. As it turns out, I'm a better friend to men than a partner. That's not to say I haven't fallen in love since Graydon, but the doubts I continued to have about being able to make a marriage work always kept me from making that final decision to marry.

Could I ever trust a lover again? I simply didn't have the tools to shed the armour I wore like a thin film surrounding my heart.

In time I adopted a motto that I believe in to this day:

Fool me once
shame on you.
Fool me twice
shame on me.

I want to ask this of you, my reader, as you ponder life with the man or woman of your dreams: Talk with each other. Listen to the goals and hopes and fears that your partner shares with you. Spend time together.

Love
with your eyes
wide open

Graydon and I talked about this and much more following the death of his second wife, Christine, and after he became a successful liver transplant survivor. Graydon nearly died during that time, and it caused me to pause and revisit our relationship, or lack of one.

As I visited Graydon one day in the Liver Transplant ICU in Toronto General hospital I vowed that, one day, we would talk. Really talk.

We exchanged many e-mails. One exercise Graydon and I put ourselves through was to share something we *should have shared* very early in our marriage. And it had to be a phone conversation. This exercise could not be put on paper, just in case some explanations were required.

I wanted to be first up.

I shared that once I heard and confirmed that Graydon was having an affair, I wished he was dead. My God, isn't that terrible? I'm shocked, even now, as I type those words.

A cheater is a cheater and should be called out. Additionally, I felt that anyone who cheats on his or her partner has already decided the marriage/partnership isn't worth fighting for. I did say to Graydon as I ended my 'secret share' that I didn't really want him dead. I only wanted him dead to me.

When I finished, Graydon laughed and asked if I had come up with the expression, 'Wanted Dead or Alive.' His humour is alive and well today in his son, James, and his grandchildren, Jalen and Lexi.

Next it was Graydon's turn. His 'share' was much deeper than mine, but I'm getting ahead of myself.

For Graydon's story, let your mind go back to the New Year of 1967.

"I'll be right back. There's something in my hockey bag for you. Find it and we'll talk later."

I would like to say we at the very least made eye contact but we did not. There was absolutely nothing romantic about Graydon's comments and no discussion followed.

Graydon reached into the back seat of his car and pulled his stinky hockey bag up and onto his seat as he got out. He couldn't flee his own car fast enough. He was off to his home in the Air Force barracks to pick something up.

This had happened before so I wasn't uncomfortable waiting in the car...no women allowed in the barracks.

I was to root through his hockey bag to find 'something' before he returned. I was beyond excited when I found the engagement ring buried in his sweaty hockey pants.

This man wanted to marry *me*?

When Graydon returned, our talk turned immediately to our wedding and not at all to whether we were suited for this huge step. We certainly did not discuss the history of the ring.

The following week I went to the jewellers, where Graydon had purchased my engagement ring. It was too big for my finger.

I knew the jeweller well and when I pulled the ring out of my bag he blurted out something like, "This ring is not for you. Is it? This is the ring I sold to Graydon Scott, I believe, but I thought it was being sent to…oh, wait…sorry, that must have been another Graydon Scott."

He knew, and so did I, that he had shared a secret Graydon wanted him to keep, especially from me.

The jeweller resized my ring and I picked it up on a day I knew he would not be in the store. I was embarrassed, and yet my thoughts were on planning my wedding, not on having a difficult discussion with my groom-to-be. In retrospect that would have been a great opportunity to open a discussion.

The beautiful engagement ring buried deep in Graydon's hockey bag was not purchased for me. He had had plans to marry someone else. And I buried that thought. Foolish me for letting that opportunity for an honest discussion pass.

I had heard rumours that Graydon was engaged or was about to become engaged to a young woman he had met and fallen in love with during his time in Europe with the Air Force's then-famous Raiders hockey team. Clearly, to my young and immature mind, this was not true.

I buried this for years, and by the time I wanted to talk about it, Graydon had re-married and I was too embarrassed to bring it up with anyone else. A story like this one surely comes with a best-before-date.

When Graydon and I finally talked about the young years we had lived decades and decades earlier, Graydon shared that his biggest secret that he wished he had never kept from me was that, in fact, he was to be engaged to someone else when he met me. There it is once more…the ring was not intended for me.

At this stage of my life, I reflect on the young woman Graydon had promised his heart to. I can't imagine how all of this would have made her feel. I'm hoping she received some form of explanation with an apology. I didn't ask.

If my relationship experiences make even one young couple stop and revisit their relationship it will have been worth 'sharing it all.'

Talk with each other. *Talk with each other.*

21: Don't hide the badass in your family

My uncle, Andy d'Entremont, and his wife, Nora, lived in Hamilton, Ontario. They are angels now, and I am proud to say I knew Uncle Andy when he was young, very much alive, single, and a badass.

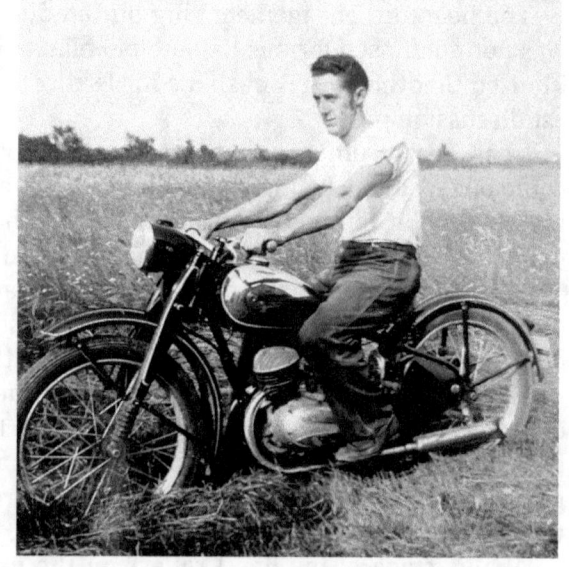

Oh, the stories he could tell. He loved to share the antics of his young life and he proudly called himself a 'biker.' If you looked closely you could also see that my uncle was a proud man.

Early in my Bell career I spent two weeks in Hamilton, Ontario for a training course. I was underage and had never set foot in a bar. That didn't stop Uncle Andy from introducing me to the bar scene in his 'hood.

During talks with my mother before heading to Hamilton, I promised her I would call her brother, and I did. I called Uncle Andy immediately upon my arrival!

We talked a bit and he asked if I knew who the Hamilton Tiger Cats were. I said of course and we spent a few minutes talking about the Canadian Football League.

Then it happened. "Would you like to meet a few of the Cats?"

"Oh My God. Would I? I sure would."

"How long are you in town?"

"Two weeks."

"In two weeks I can introduce you to every single one of the Hamilton Tiger Cats, young lady. You'll meet the whole damn team and that's a promise."

"How will I know who the single guys are?" I asked, showing just how unworldly I was.

"We can talk about that another time. We can meet them one at a time if you like. You're a pretty young thing." (Imagine if anyone said that today!)

"I'm free every evening," I said as a bit of a joke.

"Tomorrow after your class, you get your supper into your belly and then call me and I'll pick you up."

"We could have supper together. If you like."

"I don't eat much. Bad stomach. Sister Marie Rose probably told you I like my beer better than any of the food groups."

"I don't drink. Plus, my mother would kill me. Is that going to be okay with the people working at the bar? Does everyone in a bar have to drink?"

Uncle Andy had a solution for everything. "Here's what we can do to have fun together and make it all work. With every beer I buy for myself I'll buy one for you. I'll drink mine, give the empty bottle to you, and then I'll drink yours. I'll go up to the bar to replace our two beers so we don't have a waitress hovering and maybe thinking I've had too much for my own good. You can't tell anyone in the bar about our little trick, and do not tell your mother. Especially not your mother."

"*You really are a badass, then.*" I hoped I had only whispered that to myself.

"And proud of it. Should I pick you up on my bike?"

"Mom has already said *no* to that."

"Figured," Uncle Andy said with a chuckle. "What do you say we drop the 'uncle' while we're in the bar?"

"Again, my mother would kill me. Calling you my uncle is a sign of respect and that's what I'll be calling you. Mom even reminded me to always call you Uncle Andy."

"Mary Rose is right, my dear. Uncle it is!"

Uncle Andy told me he could ride his bike with the best of them. I believed him. I believe his bike was his true love at the time.

He could also balance three chairs on his chin and walk the high-wire strung tightly in his backyard. I think it served as a clothesline when he wasn't performing his act. He gave me these pictures the first evening we were together.

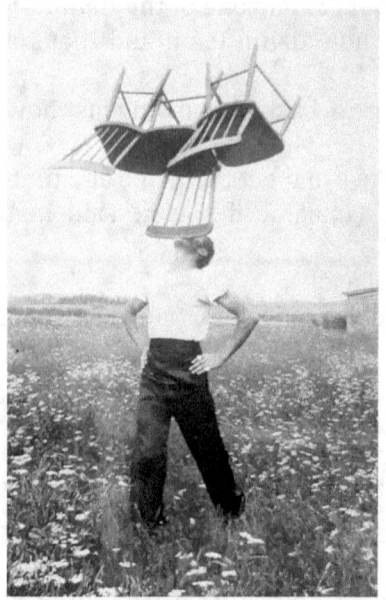 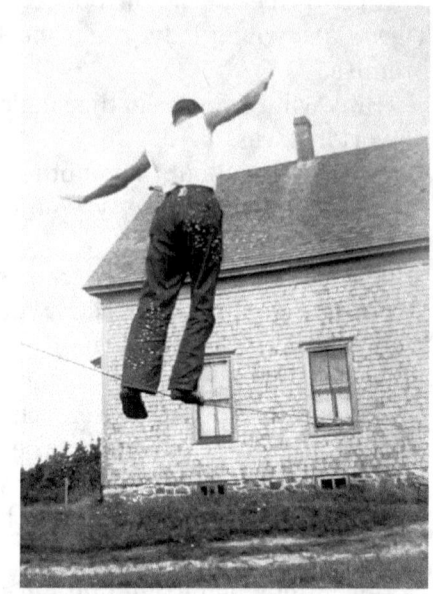

I didn't tell him that I had already seen the pictures because my mother had a copy. She was proud of her brother. He was proud of his youth captured in pictures.

I was happy to have my own copies of pictures capturing Uncle Andy's 'skills.' I recall thinking there wasn't much in the working world that required a proud young man with a chin so strong he could balance three chairs, and God knows what else. He was proud of these accomplishments and I was proud of him...a win for both of us.

We went to Uncle Andy's favourite bar *every day* after I finished my course assignment. Every day except Sunday, because, as Uncle Andy explained, "When my church-of-choice, the bar, is closed I stay home, and that only happens every Sunday."

I don't know how he did it and remained on his feet, but Uncle Andy drank his beer, and then switched his empty bottle for my untouched beer for hours at a time. I don't think anyone noticed, or cared, to be honest. We were with a rough crowd. The second Andy finished my beer he was up and at the bar in an instant for 'two more cold ones.'

He did buy a Pepsi for me at some point, but only once. It was beer or nothin!

I passed my Bell course, I did not have a drink and I believe I met each and every one of the Hamilton Tiger Cats.

Uncle Andy seemed to be proud each time he introduced me. One of the 'Cats' gave me his home phone number, and when I showed it to my uncle, he immediately tore it up.

I was proud of my badass uncle. I bet he is showing off by balancing those three chairs on his chin to make the other angels laugh.

Your thoughts:

22: Moments become memories

Keep a journal. You'll be glad you did.

I will admit, journalling is not for everyone. Case in point: I believe I had given my Nova Scotia friend, Linda Power, at least three journals as gifts before I got the message. Keeping a journal was *not* going to happen for her. Can you imagine how disappointed she must have been to receive her third journal from me? She probably felt like giving me a smack up-side-the-head with one of the journals.

Mom kept separate journals for many things:

- Changes at work that she would have to remember.
- Addresses for everyone, and for family she added birthdays and deaths.
- Personal journals that she wrote in almost every day.

When she filled one she went on to another, always dating the inside covers. She had fourteen at one point.

Do you remember having an 'autograph book' when you were young? Some would write their name and some would offer a riddle or a joke. I have autograph books that once belonged to my Aunt Ann. Her husband, Paul, gave them to me after she died. She was my mother's sister *and my God-mother*. I loved her...I still do!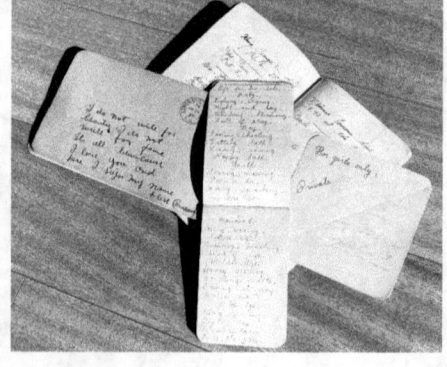

I love to read and reread Mom's journals. During the summer of 1992 we were making plans for mom to move in with me. Her journals came with her. Cancer had robbed her of so much, but it couldn't take her pride or her dignity. She packed both and moved to her new home in downtown Toronto.

Mom passed her journals on to me one snowy afternoon when we were both struggling. She was dying and I was frightened that, looking at mom, I might be looking at the mirror image of what was going to happen to me. There were moments when it was paralyzing.

Keeping the discussion on anything but cancer, I casually asked Mom what had happened to the rest of her journals. I knew there were several missing and thought she might have shared them with my sisters.

Mom's voice was strong when she told me that she had destroyed a number of journals because in those pages she was often angry and frustrated. Additionally, her journals were the only place she could whisper about the ache buried deep in her heart and the details surrounding the loss of our Wilmot home. Mom told me her dreams had died that day.

Her pride was evident as she added, and concluded, meaning I was to say no more and ask nothing more about it, "Anyway, the four of you have no business reading about my failed dreams. You have your own. Also, Carol Ann, I think I brought seven journals with me. I want to see them first because three or four of them are to be destroyed."

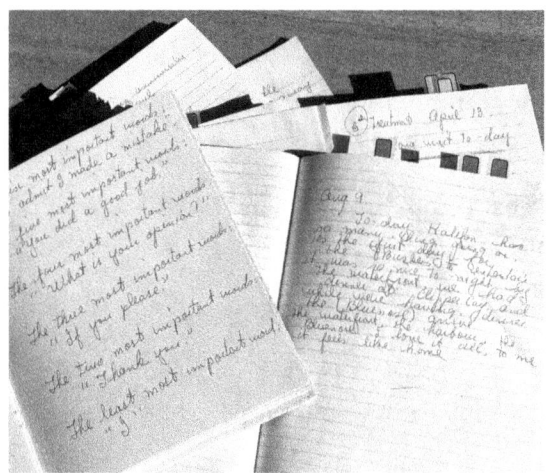

Mom smiled at that point and had more to say. "Carol Ann, I know you think other people might like to read what I have written. I don't care if you share my journals with others, but I worry that you might be disappointed with their reaction. Not everyone is going to be as interested or as proud to read my words as you are."

Through her journals, I continue to learn from my mother, many years after cancer killed her. *Cancer murdered our mother in front of our eyes.*

I have shared some of my mother's words with audiences when working as a professional speaker. Her words are a treasure-trove for me. I can't imagine anything more real than sitting down with one of her journals and talking with her as I read her written words. It's as if she is sitting beside me to this very day.

We read all seven journals, and she identified three that I was to throw away. She could tell by the date she had written before the first page. I ripped those journals to shreds in front of mom and we both laughed.

Do you journal? I would love to hear how you first began to journal and why.

This was written in mom's handwriting in one of her journals.

The 6 Most Important Words by Shane K Anderson

The 6 most important words are
I admit I made a mistake.

The 5 most important words,
You did a good job.

The 4 most important words,
What is your opinion?

The 3 most important words,
If you please.

The 2 most important words,
Thank you.

The least most important word,
I

On August 9, 1990 Mom wrote in her journal how she was feeling as we arrived in Halifax for our vacation. "Today, I'm home. Halifax has so many things going on. It's the first day for the Buskers to entertain."

Mom continued writing in her journal when we returned to our hotel room. "It was so nice tonight by the waterfront. We had dinner at the Clipper Cay [now called Salty's] and while we were having dinner, the

Bluenose arrived."

As we were getting ready for bed, mom pull out her journal one more time to write a little bit more.

> The waterfront.
> The harbour.
> The Bluenose.
> The Buskers.
> The people.
> I love it all.
> Halifax will always be home.

"Mom, I feel exactly the same way!"

Your thoughts:

23: Footprints of kindness

May 15th, 2023, I flew to Toronto from Halifax. Jalen was home from Nipissing University in North Bay, Ontario and I missed sitting down with him and having one of our heart-to-heart talks. I equally missed his sister, Lexi, and, of course, James and Tracey. I was missing Toronto friends as well, and wanted to spend a bit of time in the city so I could catch up with everyone. My plan was to return to Halifax on June 27th for at least the summer and fall. Plans don't always work out.

On June 5th I left my condo for the short walk to my dentist's office. I crossed through the Yonge/Bloor intersection with ease and turned my attention to Bloor Street West and in particular #77. I could see the door just steps ahead.

Almost there...when, for no apparent reason—no one pushed me aside or interfered with me, and the sidewalk was in pretty good shape—with no fanfare I went down. Plop on the concrete sidewalk. I heard at least two bones break and assumed I had, at the very least, broken my hip.

Actually hearing the sound of bones breaking was new to me. The pain was unbelievable.

I was instantly surrounded by airline employees, nine of them, I believe, all on a day off and out for a stroll along Bloor Street. Everyone was beyond kind and wanted to perform any number of acts of kindness for me. One took me by the arm and tried to coax me to a standing position. "Here: I'll help you up. Come on. Grab my arm."

"I need an ambulance. I'm broken."

Another flagged down a taxi. Picture his arm up and out while standing just off the sidewalk on the street shouting, "Taxi!" while I am trying to explain, one more time, "I need an ambulance. I'm broken."

One more attempt to help. "How about an Uber? Would you be more comfortable with that? I've got a direct line to my guy and he can be here in the blink of an eye."

"In the name of the Lord, please don't make me say this again. I need an ambulance. Something is broken. I heard it break."

For some reason, and I'm not sure it was a good one, my new friends decided they should get me off the sidewalk and sitting somewhere. Two kind and gentle men asked if they could pick me up. I was totally unsure how they would accomplish this but I agreed.

One held me just under the knees and the other was behind me so he put his arms gently under my arms and between the two they got me off the sidewalk.

I realized I could not put any weight on my lower body, so somewhere to sit me down became everyone's focus. I don't recall the details surrounding those minutes, and I believe I was in shock because I kept saying, "See that building at 77 Bloor Street West? It's only steps away. I am going to be so late for my appointment with my dentist. So late..."

Little did I know how late I would be.

With me perched on a slab of concrete, perhaps surrounding a tree, it was collectively decided that I really did require the assistance of ambulance services. Thank God!

One of the airline gents held my purse (which I had totally forgotten about, and my purse really does hold everything but the kitchen sink) and he, or it might have been someone else, said, "I see a policeman just across the street. I bet he could get an ambulance here faster than we could."

With that he was off to fetch the policeman.

Sean to the rescue. Currently, and maybe forever, my favourite Toronto policeman. Sean advised the airline team that they could leave me in his capable hands. They didn't need to be told a second time. I wish I had contact information for one of them so I could send a message to their group and offer a profound thank you for picking me up off a busy Toronto sidewalk in the summer of '23.

This was my first ambulance ride, and I have such respect for the job these men and women take on so they can help us in our time of need.

I asked, and then I begged, to be taken to Mount Sinai Hospital, because that's the hospital that has guided me through cancer, a chronic lung disease, a back injury that presents as a foot drop, two new knees and on and on it goes. I'm not sure how long ago this came into effect, but the ambulance attendants simply can't take you to your hospital of choice. Their system relies on the attendants to call a central number to be assigned a hospital in the area where taking one more patient is doable.

My journey took me first to a hospital on June 5th. After providing me with a drug I knew I could not tolerate, but my pain level made me believe the good emergency doctor, they sent me home.

The following day I experienced my second ambulance ride within hours of waking up, and this time I landed at St. Michael's Hospital. More testing confirmed that the first hospital was correct in diagnosing me as having fractured my tailbone, along with double fractures in my pelvis. Ouch!

All painful fractures, but the good news was that they did not require surgery. I would require lots of rest so the bones could mend, and exercises as outlined by the physical and occupational therapist who met with me in the hospital. And walking...lots of walking.

Getting my pain under control took some time and, at a time when no one wants to go to the hospital and certainly no one wants to be admitted, eleven days would pass before I arrived back home. I have only good things to say about the doctors and nurses who looked after my many roommates and me over this time.

Both doctors and nurses work hard all the time and they work long hours. They truly care for their patients. My day nurse was totally professional with me and always available when I needed her. She might need a few minutes to get to me, but she never forgot when I needed her help.

I don't know when hospitals decided that all rooms would be coed, but in all honesty I found that somewhat unsettling.

When I was first admitted and after many hours in emergency I was placed in a room around 2 am, as I recall. I could see that I had a roommate, because the curtain was drawn on my left and I could hear someone breathing. I fell asleep immediately and was startled out of a sound sleep in the darkness of night by a male voice yelling for help. He didn't stop. "Please help me. Someone help me." No one came.

When he paused to take a breath, I offered to help. "Sir, would you like me to buzz for the nurse for you?"

A very soft and different voice from the one making all the noise replied. "Who are you?"

"I'm your new roommate, sir."

"You sound like a woman."

"Good guess. Do you want me to buzz the nurse for you or not, sir?"

"You don't have to call me 'sir.' Call me 'your honour'."

My lack of sleep was apparent with my next comment. "I am not calling you 'your honour' and I am not buzzing the nurse for you either. I'm begging you to stop yelling and see if you can get some sleep."

In all of my days at St Michael's I only had one female roommate. Betsy and I became fast friends and bonded over things like the 'Red Sock Shortage' when our ward ran out of clean socks to give us. They were all red.

We visited each day and I was sad to see her leave, knowing it would be just my luck that my next roommate would be male. Sure enough. This meant there were three of us in the room...two men and me. It's not a complaint. I needed to be in the hospital and was willing to take any bed available. However, I will admit to finding it uncomfortable sharing a room with men only. When I'm hospitalized it's my preference to room with women when possible. Just sayin'. I should also state I hope to not be in a hospital bed again anytime soon!

Healing brittle bones at my age takes time, and that's a dance that has forced me to slow down.

What I would say to women my age is that every single time you walk out of your home, remember to watch you step and take good care of your health. You don't want to be one of the statistics that show that a growing number of geriatric women who fall do not get to go back to their home. They require long-term care, and in some cases that might mean forever. The doctors reviewed these statistics with me before I was discharged and I found it all too close to home and frightening.

In my case I had everything working against me. I presented as a geriatric female with osteoporosis and 'of slight stature', as one doctor put it. My fracture clinic doctor suggested healing might take a year or, in my case, longer.

June 26 was a date I didn't want to miss as I and a number of friends had a pre-arranged date with Dorothy Dunbar. Most of us knew each other from our Bell days, and we were all friends with Dorothy. Friends making time for friends in this busy world can be difficult to accomplish, and a gift we give to each other. Annually we all show up at Dorothy's doorstep. We have a wonderful time catching up on everything Bell, but not before sharing everything in our personal lives.

This was my first outing since my fall, and it gave me a chance to test my walking-with-my-walker skills. Jo-Ann Luciani picked me up and made sure I was delivered back to my condo with no additional broken bones at day's end. I often caught her 'keeping an eye on me', and I fear she would have had a much better time if I had stayed home. Jo-Ann did not want me to fall on her watch. I appreciated her help that day so much.

I was not able to fly back to Halifax until August 9th, and I brought two of my three fractures home with me.

24: Know when to be 'done'

This chapter is dedicated to the memory of my Middleton Regional High School friend, Sharon Seamone.

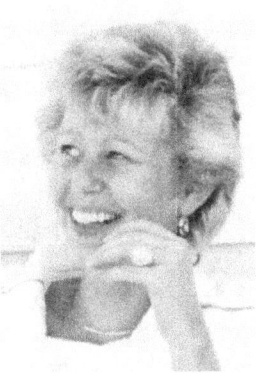

I often share this particular quote with cancer patients: 'Know when to be done.' When you feel you can't take any more chemo, or maybe it's ra-diation or it could be both, speak up or have someone else do it for you. If you're scheduled for fifteen, ten, or five cycles of a specific treat-ment and you're at the point of thinking the treatment, not the cancer, might be what kills you, speak up. Your body. Your decision.

I hear patients say, "I hate to be a quitter, but my body can't take one more chemotherapy treatment." Listen to me, please. *This does not, e-v-e-r make you a quitter. Not ever!*

I believe that sometimes you *just have to be done*. Not mad. Not upset. Just done. It's never lost on me how many cancer patients, or families of these patients, will understand what I'm saying before those who have never had to step inside an oncology ward. Survivors have been there. They've seen what treatments can do to their body. To their mind. To their family.

~

I have met many very special friends as a result of my Comfort Heart Ini-tiative. If they have a Comfort Heart, they are likely to be in touch. Most I have never met in person. To date, this little pewter heart has raised one and one half million dollars for the Canadian Cancer Society.

Sharon owned a Comfort Heart. She also purchased several for her family and friends some years before cancer knocked on her door.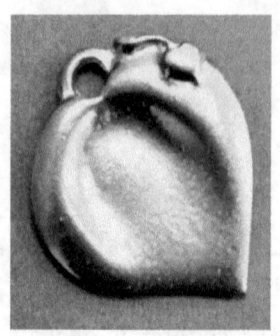

I am left with the memory of a dear friend who repeatedly suffered the body blows that come with both chemo and radiation, *administered at the same time and in heavy doses*, because the cancer within her ravaged her body from the inside out. Sharon died on January 18, 2023 because of cancer and possibly repeated treatments, at seventy-six years young.

Her desire to live and stay in this world was the strongest I have ever seen in anyone. She would repeatedly say to her oncology team, "There must be something else. I'll take it all. Please find something else. I'm begging you. You have to keep me alive."

Sharon and I had many discussions about who would determine when her 'done' should happen.

Would it be her doctors and specialists who would tell her on what date her last chemo would be, when her last radiation treatment would be?

Would her body dictate her last treatment?

Would her mind aid in helping her make these decisions prior to the final dates as struck by her oncologists?

Sharon lived her retirement years in Truro, Nova Scotia. She made friends, had a doctor she respected and so many specialists both in Truro and in Halifax. She was 100% supportive of every medical decision made on her behalf.

The time came when Sharon was hospitalized because she was so weak and sick from her treatments, and I'm sure from the spread of cancer as well. We talked about all of this and, to be honest, I was certain she would be done at that point and would return to Truro and her puppy.

Not a chance. Sharon called and, in a barely-there voice, told me that she would stay in the hospital and finish her radiation treatments. Her will to live for many more years outweighed her struggle with treatments. Her body almost gave up when she had finished her fifth of the seven remaining radiation treatments. Then and only then was she done.

It was, and is always, a daunting decision to make.

Sharon's palliative care at home in Truro was flawless. She had three skilled ladies at her door every day. It seemed every time I called her, someone was there to help her. Friends, former partners and family were also there for her.

A lifetime ago, while attending Middleton Regional High School, and specifically on the basketball court, Sharon and I forged a friendship that was meant to last a lifetime. She was a gifted athlete and in excellent shape. I wasn't too shabby either.

We lost and found our friendship over the years and every time we reconnected our feet were firmly planted in friendship for a lifetime and beyond.

A basketball game is in our future. We agreed to a match on the court.

We laughed and we cried each time we talked. And, it wasn't morbid at all. We were realistic, or so we thought, as we firmed up a plan for me to drive from Halifax to Truro and pull into her driveway! A road trip would follow. Sharon always asked me to wait until she felt better and she would let me know when that day arrived.

Sometimes you just have to be done.
Not mad, not upset. Just done!

When Sharon was released from a Halifax hospital, she was transferred by ambulance to the Truro hospital where she would take endless physiotherapy sessions because she could not walk, couldn't sit up in bed. She was too weak to feed herself and couldn't get to the bathroom on her own. In summary, Sharon was a mess. She would always say, "I'm a mess but there is a basketball court in my future."

International Women's Day, March 8th, 2022 Sharon was happy to be at home, learning how to walk and talk and feed herself all over again.

International Women's Day 2023 told a very different story. My friend, Sharon, was gone from this earth. Cancer took her body limb by limb, organ by organ, and finally it invaded her brain.

Murdered by cancer.

I will never forget you, Sharon Seamone. I bet you have already formed a basketball team in heaven. Use a sub for one of the spots on your team. Keep it for me. We will play basketball again!

25: The lucky ones grow old

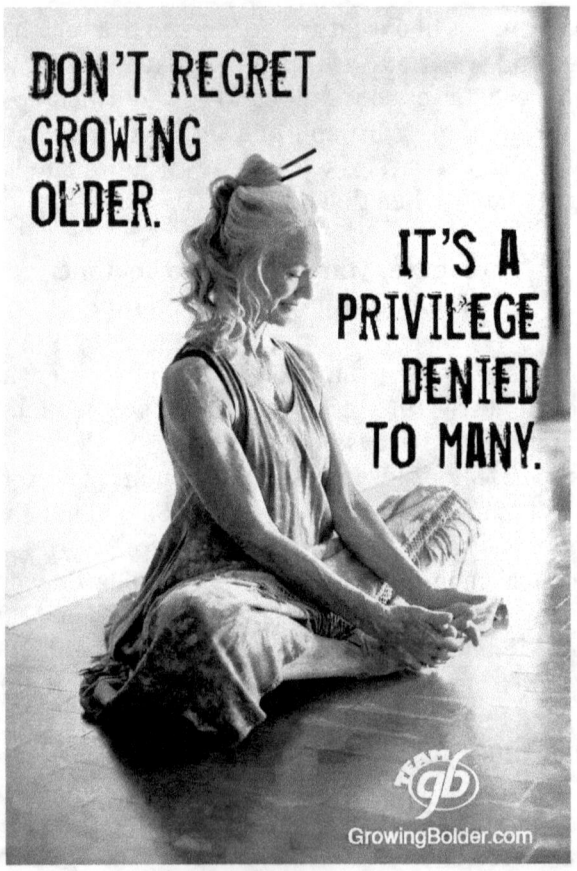

We were all young once.

My mother told me a story that, initially, I found hard to believe. She felt that after she turned sixty-five she was made to feel invisible. She had examples.

One sunny and warm day, when mom took the bus to the Scarborough Town Centre, she had a question for the driver. She had difficulty getting his attention, so she quietly deposited her ticket and found a seat. He didn't hear a word my mother spoke and he didn't see her because there was a pretty young girl directly behind mom. He even addressed the young woman as a 'pretty young thing.'

It's possible mom took it all wrong, or didn't hear the entire conversation, or didn't try hard enough to capture and keep the bus driver's attention, but none of that changed the way the bus driver and the situation made her feel...invisible. We are all entitled to our own feelings. They belong to us.

I was convinced Mom misunderstood the situation...until it happened to me. I was made to feel invisible in a similar manner and I was not yet 60! Given that this did not happen to mom until she was past sixty-five was not lost on me.

I'll apologize to mom for not believing her when we next meet. She's saving me a seat in heaven. No ticket required.

Today I celebrate everything, including every birthday I am fortunate enough to have. During Hurricane Lee in 2023, my three sisters and I were together to celebrate two milestones. Lois had turned 80 and the baby of the family, Connie, turned 70 in October. Not lost on us is the fact that we are still Mary's four girls. I'm so thankful.

Your thoughts:

26: Keep your COVID mask

I firmly believe masks will be part of our lives forever. They certainly will be part of mine. At the very least, keep a mask in your pocket 'just in case.'

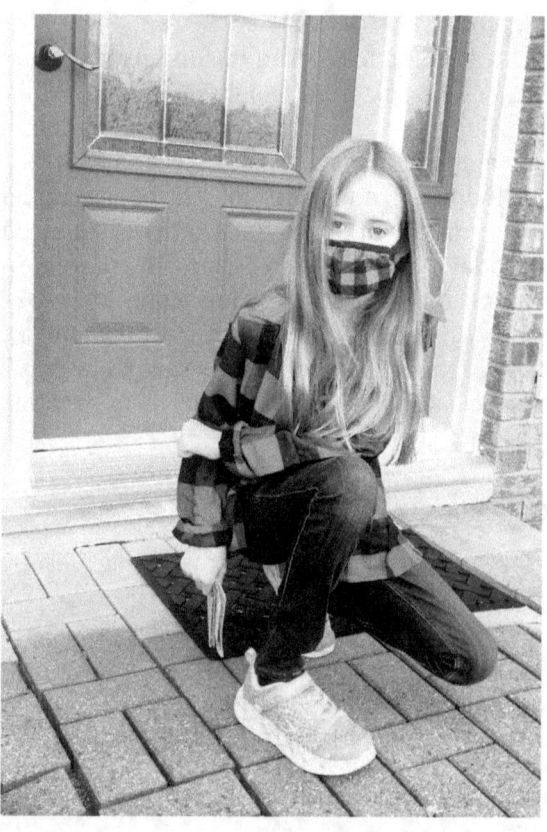

This picture of Lexi was taken on her first school day in grade five. Lexi is a people person and an artist. She is intelligent, inclusive, bold, brave, funny, creative and beautiful. She is resolved to wear a mask when she must and if she's unsure she has parents who are dialed into the risks of wearing or not wearing a mask, so either way Lexi can be confident as she heads off to school each day.

COVID knocked us down and too many people died because of this pandemic. Don't let your guard down. Keep your mask handy and wear it to stay safe.

27: Exercise

I worked out at Gold's Gym in downtown Toronto at 6 am before going to the office five days a week, and longer on weekends. Post retirement from Bell, I kept at it...until one day the body looking back at me in the mirror was not the one I envisioned en route to the gym.

I didn't see it coming. How could my body betray me when I had worked so hard to keep everything where it once was? And as tight as it once was. I hate it when that happens!

Today my favourite exercise is walking on the boardwalk along the Halifax harbour, and through Yorkville in Toronto. My fracture clinic doctor suggested I forget all of the other exercises I was doing and walk... simply walk every day of my life.

I have had my own take on different fads through the years for exercise purposes. Walking, running, stretching, yoga, Pilates, Jane Fonda, Tony Little, weight lifting, etc. I try to add an exercise or two to my daily walks. I struck a deal with myself when I stopped being an exercise fanatic that, in addition to walking each day, I would exercise while watching *The Young and the Restless* five days a week. Works for me.

I'm proud of my battle scars and I reflect on every scar I have earned while I walk. It's a great time to evaluate your mental health in particular. Every day I appreciate that I'm still alive and can look at my scars.

Since my last non-fiction book, I have had surgery to remove cataracts from both eyes and I have two new knees. My bookends will forever be breast cancer x 2.

Exercise.
Listen to your body.
Don't ignore health related warning signs.
And walk...every day that you can.

28: Check your expression

The expression-connection was one I learned in the summer of 1978, when I reported for work at 393 University Avenue in downtown Toronto to begin a brand-new opportunity with Bell.

One of my peers in my new work-world offered to 'show me the ropes', and I appreciated him for it.

The first thing I learned from this manager, as we entered a conference room to give a presentation, was to check my expression. His had turned sour.

Before turning the projector on (it was 1978, remember...he carried the projector and I carried the view graphs) he offered a big sigh, followed by, "I haven't had much time to put this together for you gentleman, so I'll apologize now for my errors or omissions."

Any time someone begins a presentation, or even a conversation at home, with a big sigh, rarely will this be a good-news story. For many the sigh is nothing more than a bad habit...check yours.

The only expression this manager offered was indeed a negative one. He was almost asking his boss and his boss's boss to watch for his mistakes throughout his presentation.

I wanted to ask about his turn of expression when we were on the elevator going back to our offices far away from the ivory tower, however, since he was supposed to be teaching me I decided to keep my mouth shut. In fact, to him, it seemed that it had 'gone pretty good upstairs with the boys.'

I learned to pick a time and a place to offer a sigh, so I did learn something from the presentation.

This manager was gone a short time after our first encounter. I would learn that his 'performance', as it was called back then, was less than stellar. In fact, it was less than satisfactory and this had been the case for some time. A 'less than satisfactory performance' gets you noticed for all the wrong reasons. Often all it gets you is 'gone'!

Your expression is your most important garment.
Ensure your expression
Represents the real you.

Your thoughts:

29: How will you be remembered?

**Before they care how much you know,
they need to know how much you care.**

A friend shared the above quote with me many years ago, and it has stuck with me. It's true. I believe soft skills should be part of the high school curriculum.

You can leave university with any number of degrees on your office wall, but not respecting your employees, peers and 'higher ups' will cause you any number of problems. Your staff will leave you and go to a company where they know they will feel respected and valued as members of the team.

I'm not necessarily proud of the fact that, regardless of the job I had at any given time, I was on a first name basis with the night cleaning staff. I did nothing more than ask their name, introduce myself and ensure they understood they could enter my office when they were scheduled to do so. I did not want to delay their work schedule. It must be hard to work nights at any job, and I suspect cleaning offices is not always fun. It's the little things...

Maya Angelou has touched many of us. She has a better way with words than I do...

**I've learned that people will forget what you said,
people will forget what you did,
but people will never forget
how you made them feel.**

30: Life is not fair

My initial intent was to simply say it again.

> *Life is not fair.*
> **Accept it.**
> **Move on.**

We all experience unfairness at one time or another...and it's easy to get into the mindset that the 'unfairness' only happens to us. It happens to everyone and, no, it's not always fair.

There are endless examples of this...

An employee is unjustly fired.

My Leafs fail to win the Stanley Cup.

A child receives a cancer diagnosis.

A couple is unable to have a baby.

You lose a loved one at a young age.

Your best jewellery has been stolen.

You learn your partner is a cheater.

A grandchild is born with severe disabilities.

Add to this list your own examples of life smacking you upside the head. It doesn't hurt our children and grandchildren to know that we, too, have had disappointments and flat tires as we travel life's highway.

We all have to understand that...

Life

is

not

fair.

Your thoughts:

31: Maturity wears many different faces

Maturity is when

> you know
> the other person
> is lying
> but
> you smile anyway
> and let it go.

We've all been there. 'Letting it go' is not always an easy thing to do. Maturity guides you if you allow it to happen. David Bowie calls it 'aging.'

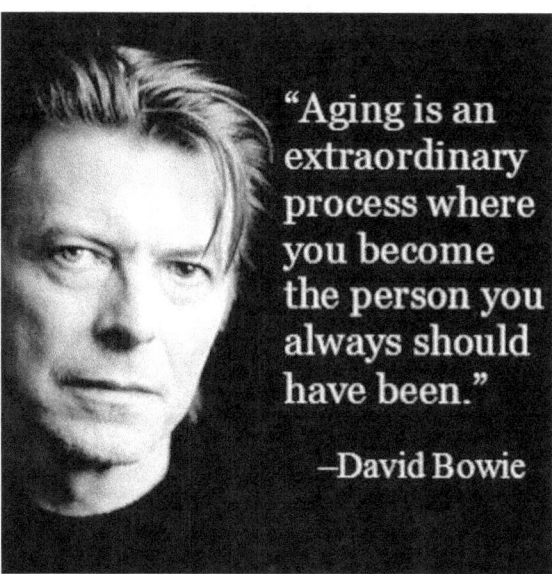

"Aging is an extraordinary process where you become the person you always should have been."

–David Bowie

32: Leave your own footprints of kindness for others to discover

There is much to be said about small gestures...an offer of help, or being present in someone's life when it's not expected. Drop off a few groceries because you had to go to the grocery store anyway. A gentle tap on the shoulder speaks volumes.

> **There is a stranger**
> **somewhere**
> **who still remembers you**
> **because you were kind to them**
> **when no one else was.**

The above quote reminds me of a friend of mine, Nancy Stoddart, who leaves her personal footprints of kindness every single day. Nancy is the person who helped *that* stranger. And the person she helps will forever remember Nancy.

As of April, 2022, Nancy had made and given away over *five thousand masks*. She covered all costs herself. Nancy also makes 'grippers' to help open that pesky jar of jam that just won't open.

One afternoon Nancy and I were running a few errands, so stopping here and there. I watched her reaction as a lady passing by said, 'Love your mask.'

Nancy immediately reached into her bag and pulled out a new mask and asked if the lady would like to have it. We were still in the parking lot! The exchange took less than a minute.

Nancy saw a young woman with a child who were struggling with something the child wanted opened, 'right now', so Nancy to the rescue with a 'gripper.'

On to the next store, where we were lined up to pay for our purchases when Nancy witnessed a young woman taking things out of her cart, quite possibly because she knew she wouldn't have enough money to pay for everything. Sure enough, in her handbag Nancy had a couple of coupons that might be helpful to this lady.

She approached her and in a hushed voice said she had some coupons that were due to expire soon and she knew she wouldn't make it to this particular store in time to use them. "If you could use them I would appreciate it. I would hate for them to expire and therefore benefit no one."

Imagine how appreciative this woman was. Nancy allowed this young woman to feel that she was helping Nancy, not the other way around. That's a gift.

Nancy is the stranger who cares enough to make a difference in the life of another stranger. I believe there is never a day that this woman doesn't help one or two or a few people.

When I flew to Halifax from Toronto in August, 2023, after having the fall I mentioned earlier, Nancy picked me up at the airport and delivered me to my condo downtown. None of my friends, Nancy included, like driving downtown because of the construction and the abundance of cars on the streets, but she made an exception this time. I was hobbling along with a walker that I was still getting used to.

Not only did Nancy deliver me safely, but she had a trunk full of frozen meals for me. I lost count of how many things she had ready for me but, trust me, I had homemade food for weeks.

Your thoughts:

33: What does 'just' mean to you?

The way we use the word 'just,' in most cases, is nothing more than a bad habit we develop throughout the years.

You can have a bit of fun with young children in your life when they call you and say, "Hi Nana, it's *just* me." Teach them to introduce themselves with pride. "Hi Nana, it's me!"

If they are calling to chat with you, teach them to not use the following expressions...

> Hi, it's ~~just~~ me...
>
> Nana it's ~~just~~ me. I'm selling...
>
> I was ~~just~~ thinking...
>
> I was ~~just~~ wondering if...
>
> Nana, I ~~just~~ wanted to ask...

As a family, when you're all in the same room, see who can go the longest without using the word 'just' in any conversation. Make a memory with it.

I have found that grandchildren, especially as they enter their teenage years, will thank you for this tip. If you're able, have fun with it, and it can be a teachable moment that can be passed on and on and on.

You are never 'just' anyone. You can add to your confidence by deleting the word from your memory bank.

34: Let others gossip without you

I'm sure almost everyone would agree they have lent an ear to gossip at least a few times during their life. Gossip usually involves love, relationships, sex and other issues that are not always talked about in public. It often causes pain and humiliation for the person it is about.

There will always be people who gossip with no thought of how it might impact the individual…especially in this social media world. I'm glad I am not a young adult today. Someone they will never know could capture their every move.

There are any number of reasons why individuals will spread rumours or engage in gossip. It might be for what they see as appeal, to gain power, to get revenge, to feel better, to feel accepted and perhaps even to relieve boredom.

I once stood in a buffet line in Halifax when a friend pointed to a man standing a dozen people ahead of us and said, "See that guy? He was charged with rape." This was almost said with pride. I asked if he was convicted. No, he was not. I did not need that information in the first place and was left to try to erase the discussion from my memory.

Imagine how that man would have felt if he had overheard this woman proudly telling me something about him that I did not need to know. I believe he would feel he had indeed been convicted in public opinion polls. He perhaps realized he would be gossiped about for the rest of his natural life and always with this as the lead discussion.

If someone is charged and convicted, their life implodes. However, if a charge is dropped because there wasn't enough evidence to go to court, this is very different and the discussion should cease at that time. 'Charges dropped' is supposed to mean *end of*.

There are times when a charged man who has that charge dropped still suffers more than those incarcerated. Whatever the reason, don't be part of it. One rumour leads to another and another and another. Each story is a bit more juicy than the last.

Gossip is exhausting and unnecessary. I remember vividly engaging in, and originating, gossip during my younger years. Some from my Business office service representative days in North Bay would likely say I 'got what I deserved' in the end. The upside is that I did learn the lesson. Fortunately, I had managers at work who cared about me and let me know the damage my gossip was causing.

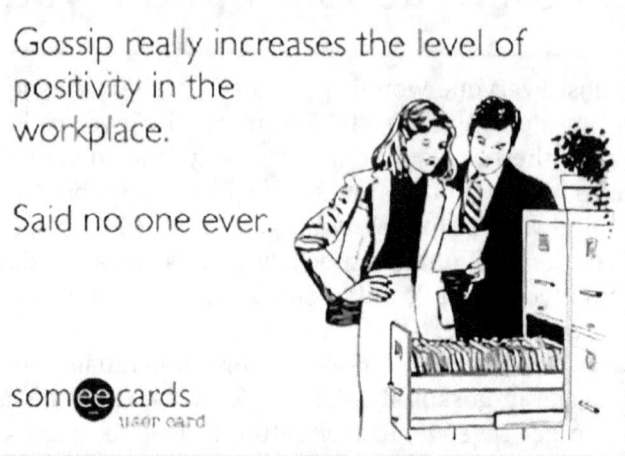

Your thoughts:

35: Don't look down on others

Perhaps, at some point in your life, you have looked down on those who...

> Service your car,
> Pour your coffee when you're on the run,
> Clean your home because you choose not to,
> Paint your home because you're too busy at the office,
> Empty the garbage bins you leave at the end of your driveway...

Everyone deserves to be treated with respect. Everyone.
Looking down on someone makes you unattractive to others. A select number of individuals are in your world for a reason. *You pay them to make your day a bit easier.*

Be kind. Be caring. Say...

> 'I appreciate you.'
> 'Thank you for your time.'
> 'You have made my day a bit easier to manage, thank you.'
> 'If you couldn't do your job, I couldn't do mine.'

Jot down a few examples of people from your own memory bank that you could share with your children, or grandchildren, showing their kindness, their caring for others. Your discussion can make a difference in someone's life.

36: Siblings are special

I have three sisters and I am forever grateful that we are all in good health...*relatively good health.*

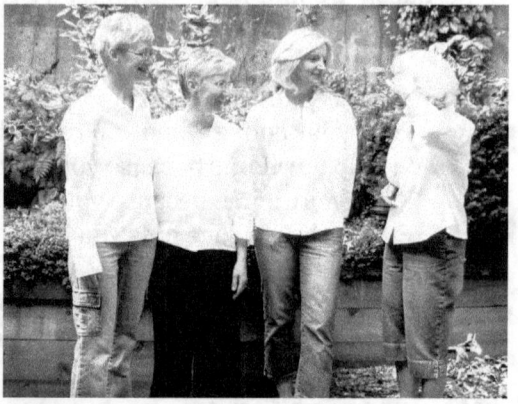

I love this picture because, on the right, Lois is using the same gesture that mom used for one of two reasons, either to keep the sun out of her eyes or to let us know that 'enough is enough.'

Thank you to our professional photographer, Sue Mills, who captured us in both photos.

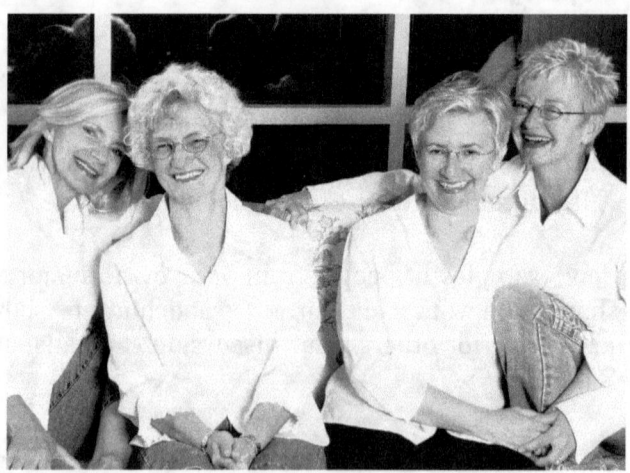

My lovely sister pack! Me with Lois, Lorraine and Connie.

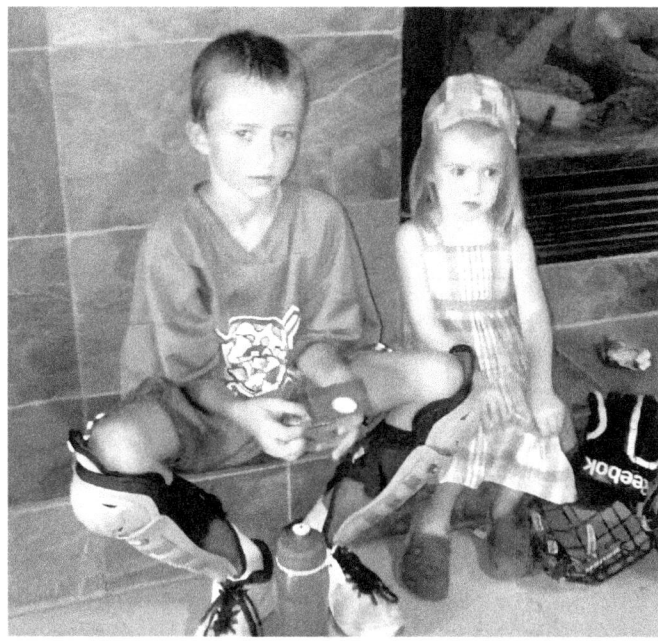

Jalen and Lexi are also siblings and this is one of my absolute favourite pictures of them together. It comes with a true story about their connection.

Jalen's ball-hockey team had just lost the championship game in a weekend tournament. Feeling totally sad and almost in tears, Jalen sat alone. He didn't want anyone to sit with him and he didn't want to talk.

His sister loved everything about any tournament her brother played in. And she equally loved her brother. Lexi brought her dolls and her doll carriage to the games, and played with her own 'hockey friends' who were the younger sisters of many of the hockey players. Every now and then she could be heard shouting, "Go Jalen. Go Jalen." On occasion, she brought, and used, her pompoms.

Suddenly, on this particular day, seeing her brother looking so sad, Lexi dropped what she was doing and went to Jalen's side. Without saying a word and wearing her sad/mad face Lexi sat as close to her brother as she could. She was unsure why they were so sad but she was putting on a good face, don't you think?

That's what siblings do. Do you have siblings? Do your children have siblings? Make a note of stories that make you smile. Share those smiles with your family.

37: Volunteer

You are never too young to lend a hand.

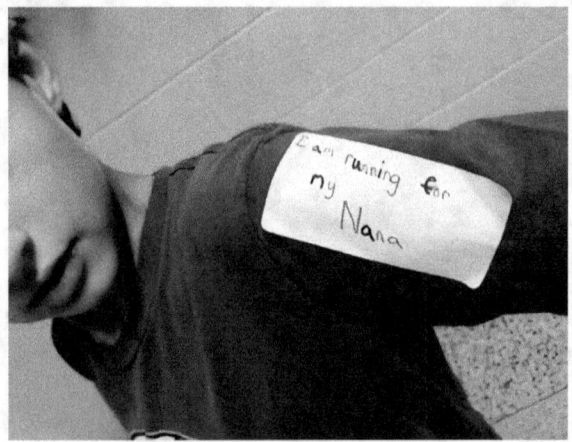

I chose to be involved in volunteering while I was with Bell. However; it became a bit more difficult once I retired. No computer, no printer, etc. And few contacts.

It didn't take me long to gather what I would need. At the time, I could see how difficult it might be for many who wanted to set up their own fundraising effort and didn't have the resources available to me.

I had just retired from Bell and the then-President, John McLennon, and Ruth Foster ensured that Bell covered the cost of purchasing Comfort Hearts to be used in the initial marketing program. Bell also covered the cost of brochures, and bookmarks given out at my memoir launch with a Comfort Heart attached to each.

I partnered with the Canadian Cancer Society and the Comfort Heart Initiative, in my mother's memory, was born.

My grandchildren run to honour the memory of Terry Fox and for their Nana who has beaten cancer. Twice! This was as personal for them as it was for me. When you see your grandson with a sticker on his arm saying, 'I'm running for my Nana' and at a later date your granddaughter, with a sticker on her sleeve saying, 'I'm running for Terry Fox and for my Nana,' it fills your heart with so much pride and gratitude.

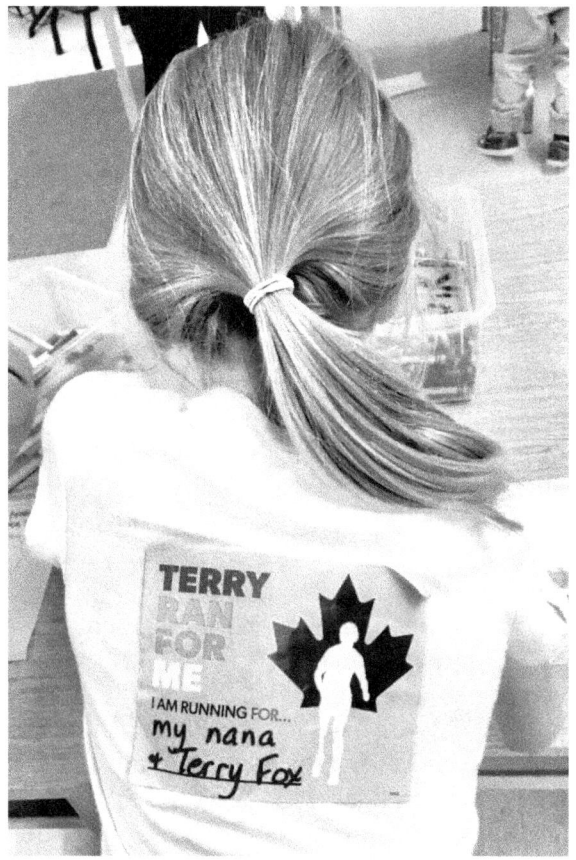

38: Acknowledge family dynamics

When I hear someone say, 'I have become successful *in spite of* my family,' I wonder if they really mean what they say.

Whenever possible, I try to turn that attitude around, using myself as the example. 'If I have become successful at all, it's not *in spite of* my family. It is *because of* my family...my entire family.

We learn from every person who comes into our lives. When it's a bad experience, it is still a learning opportunity if we allow it to be. I believe it is important to not turn your back on anyone from your family. I do know that's not always possible, but it's always worth one more effort. It goes back to my belief that we could all be nice...twice.

Without naming names, when my memoir came out, one of my book signings was at the Inside Story in Greenwood, NS, where a rather awkward situation presented itself. I was busy signing books and talking with friends and family when the manager of the bookstore came over to me.

"Carol Ann, is there any chance you know the individual who has climbed into our window display area? He is attempting to remove the large poster of your book cover that we have in our main window. I have asked him to step down but he won't. I don't think he was listening to me at all. He's using some sort of a pocketknife to loosen the tape keeping the poster in our window."

In a whisper she continued, "We have called Mall Security, and if they can't get him out of there they will call the police."

Looking over to the window, I replied, "Ah, yes, I do know that man. I will deal with him right away."

I asked those waiting in line to give me a second to deal with a family emergency. Chuckles all around. I believe they were enjoying the entertainment.

Closing in on the area that would allow me to lean into the window display, I am ashamed to admit I assumed he was drunk.

I know it would be more colourful if I gave you his full name but I am not going to do that.

"Hey, what are you doing? You're making a scene and I need you to stop it and get out of that window."

I was not expecting his reply. "This is your picture and by God I'm having this poster."

I could see he was using a small knife that he most likely had in his pocket for dozens of years and today he was using it on my poster.

I didn't get any closer to him in case he turned on me. It wouldn't have been the first time.

Trying to find a resolution I offered an alternative. "I'll tell you what I will do...just for you. How would you like a brand new poster with no tape around the edges? I'll even sign it for you, if you like. But in return you must get out of that window box right now. And, you might consider leaving the Mall."

That seemed to do the trick. I watched him fold the knife, return it to his pocket and proceed to jump down to floor level. As he leaned in to whisper in my ear I was ashamed that I had assumed he was drunk. I couldn't smell alcohol on his breath...not a smidge.

"Hey, don't write on my poster. *You'll ruin it*. I don't need you to mark on it at all. I know who you are."

Good enough. He got his poster sent directly to his home, compliments of my publisher, ECW Press in Toronto.

Your thoughts:

39: I hope you dance

When you get the chance to sit out
or dance
I hope you dance!

...from Lee Ann Womack

I miss having a dance partner.

To this day I dance alone and in every room of my condo, but it's not the same. In fact, for years, I have shared with close friends that I have missed dancing more than sex.

Brian Bastedo and I dated for a period of time and he did sign us up for ballroom dance lessons. However, he did this *after* we had broken up and, as much as I would have loved to take dance lessons with Brian, it was not meant to be.

Dance like no one is watching.

Because they're not.

They're checking their phones.

Graydon and I danced often when our marriage was young. I loved it so much. We would go dancing with our good friends, Beth and Jim Filipov. Beth and I would joke that Graydon and Jim spent more time talking with each other than they did with us whenever we were all on the dance floor. And we were on the dance floor at least once a week. To add to that, Beth and I also decided that when the four of us were on the dance floor it must have looked to others that she and I were dancing together and Graydon and Jim were dancing with each other.

I can still see Graydon's smile during those early days of love, dancing, romance and dreams. This I keep in my memory bank!

I hope *you* dance!

Your thoughts:

40: Learn to like your own company

In my entire life I did not live alone until my son moved out. I lived in Wilmot with my family, followed by a huge move to the big city of North Bay, Ontario. I have moved well over a dozen times since my North Bay days, where I lived with my Aunt Edith, Uncle Ken, and sons Chuck, Brian and Gary.

I love living alone. Friends have asked if I'm ever lonely and I respond with honesty. The short answer is yes, I sometimes feel lonely. *However, the price I pay for being alone when I want to be alone is that I am also alone when I would rather not be alone.*

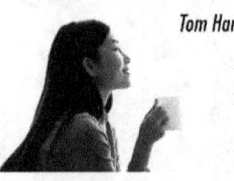

> ## Some people don't understand that sitting in your own house alone in peace, eating snacks and minding your own business is priceless.
>
> *Tom Hardy*

I'm fortunate to have a wonderful family and friends whom I cherish.

I do like my own company. And you should, too.

After a certain age I think we deserve to do what makes us happy. In my case, writing plays a big part in my daily life. I think it would be harder to concentrate on the current project as much and for as long as I need to, if I lived with other people. I'm passionate about writing...this book is my fifth non-fiction. I currently have five novels published as well.

When I first began writing fiction I found it difficult. Paradise d'Entremont was the only fully-rounded character I had for years. Now, thanks in large part to my editor, Andrew Wetmore, I have learned to slow down and let my characters take the lead. They sometimes lead me to a different plot for the chapter than the one I'm working on at the moment. In one case, the final sequence in a novel changed course completely about thirty pages prior to the end of the book. I did not see that coming!

Talking about being alone and sometimes being lonely can be a difficult conversation to have. Make your notes here if you like.

My mother, especially during her retirement years, enjoyed her alone time. Often she spent those moments reading one of her many books, making notes when she finished and giving the book a passing or a failing grade.

Mom's journals recorded her thanks for so many things. She moved to Ontario, having lived her entire life in Nova Scotia, and noted in her journal that she was celebrating six years since she left her beloved Nova Scotia. I love this note.

41: Never give up

For reasons I do not remember, I was asked to memorize and recite a poem during one of my 'graduations' at Wilmot School...possibly once I had learned to manage my stuttering, which would have been during grade five or six.

Looking back, it seems like a rather serious poem to ask a student to memorize, but I didn't see it that way. I was proud to do it. My teacher knew about my difficult relationship with my father and this might have been her way of 'talking to me about it' without talking about it. Does that make sense?

My teacher, with my mother's help, took me from a stuttering young student who couldn't read aloud during class because of this communication disorder, to a student who was proud to step on to the school stage and face all the Wilmot and area students and parents.

I'm certain this poem was called 'Don't You Quit''. Following is only a small part of the poem. I do not know the author's name.

> Don't give up
> When things go wrong
> as they sometimes will,
> when the road you're trudging
> seems all uphill,
> when funds are low
> and debts are high,
> and you want to smile
> but you have to sigh,
> when life is pressing
> you down a bit,
> rest,
> if you must
> but don't you quit.

Both my mother and my teacher had tears in their eyes as I took a bow while the audience applauded. This was the beginning of my love of public speaking.

Your thoughts:

42A: Cancer is a beast

This chapter is dedicated to the memory of my dear friend Kathy Service.

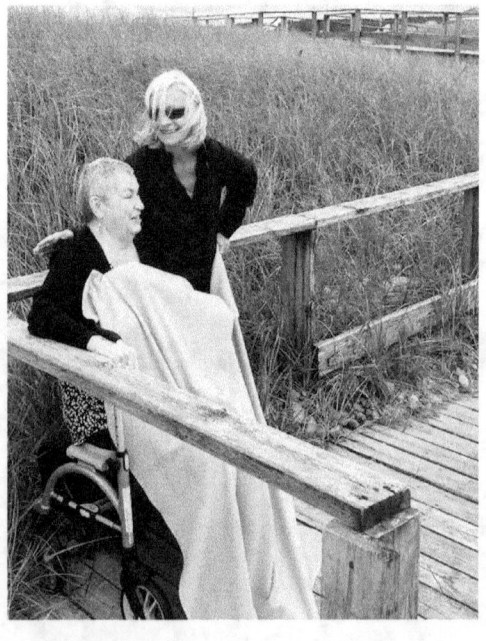

Kathy's daughters, Heather and Shannon, snapped a number of pictures of the two of us engaged in conversation at Lawrencetown Beach, Nova Scotia. This is the last picture I have of us together, and it carries one of my most treasured memories.

Brain cancer, glioblastoma to be specific, did not stop Kathy from visiting Nova Scotia one more time. In this photo she was worried that I was going to be cold. She removed her jacket, insisted that I put it on, and only then did she ask me to help her pull her blanket up over her body to keep warm.

"How will I explain to your daughters that I needed your jacket because I was cold?" I was laughing as I asked the question. Additionally, Kathy's granddaughter, Hannah, was part of the team and to her young mind why on earth would I be wearing her Nana's jacket?

"I'm anxious to see that so I leave it firmly in your hands." Humour was still evident in this vibrant woman loved by so many.

Brain cancer robbed us of this kind and caring woman, who battled the beast for just over a year.

Kathy and I met in the late 60s in North Bay, Ontario. Our individual lives were very busy and there were long stretches of time over the years when we didn't see each other at all. And yet our bond was unbreakable.

When my dear friend took her last trip around the sun, we didn't talk about cancer exclusively. There were days when we didn't talk about her health at all.

I always tried to take my lead from Kathy. She talked a lot about her son and two daughters and all that she would miss in their lives. She had hoped to have more time with her children and her grandchildren.

Hannah was Kathy's youngest granddaughter. One of the many reasons she wanted to bring Hannah along on her last trip to Nova Scotia was that she wanted them to make more memories together...just the two of them.

Kathy, her husband, Bill, and often the entire family could be seen at a Jays game.

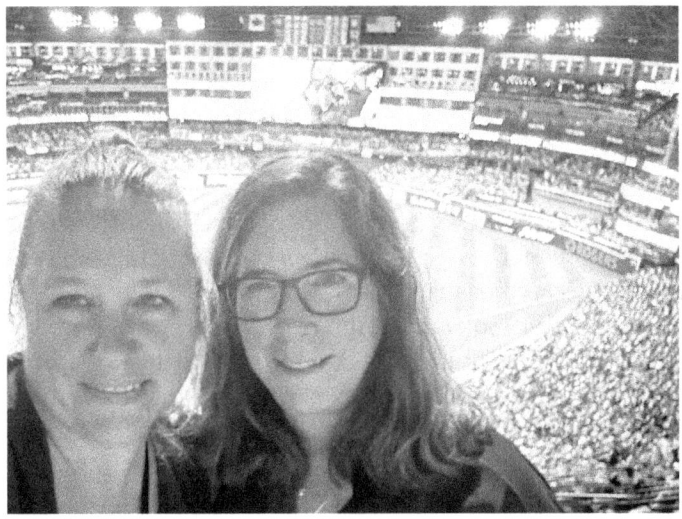

This is a very recent picture of Heather and Shannon, taken at a Jays game in early October, 2023. They were celebrating Shannon's birthday. I miss the connection to Kathy's daughters that I enjoyed while Kathy was alive. I need to do better going forward to restore our friendship. I promised Kathy that I would keep in touch with her family. That's on me. I'll fix this!

During her retirement years, Kathy worked and travelled with special needs adults. She very quickly taught me to drop the word 'needs.' I can hear her now: "Carol Ann, they are not 'special needs' people. They are 'special' people."

I met a number of her new friends and they were indeed special. They had so much love and respect for 'Miss Kathy.'

Using the term 'special' rather than 'special needs' really is a kinder way for all of us to show greater compassion towards others. I thanked Kathy more than once for teaching me this lesson.

Kathy and I talked about some of the things said to us about our cancer experiences, beginning when we were first diagnosed. For the most part we agreed it's difficult to find the right words, and as a result people may misspeak without intending to. They hope the right words will come to them when they open their mouth…

That's okay, by the way. Speak from your heart and move forward from there. It's totally fine to say, "I don't know what to say," when you meet someone who is struggling with cancer or with any illness.

I captured my own thoughts about what you should not say to a cancer patient some years ago, in my book *Lessons Learned Upside the Head*. With Kathy's help, I have revisited this topic here.

Kathy was receiving radiation treatments for her brain cancer, and during the week she stayed at the Princess Margaret Lodge in downtown Toronto. Her family and friends ensured she was never alone during these long days and nights.

On the night I had the privilege of occupying the other single bed in her room, I was given a 'check in' time and was told not to have too much to eat during the day because Kathy was taking me out to dinner. *This lady with brain cancer took me to dinner.*

We walked to the restaurant and, while it is indeed very close to the Lodge, I was nervous about Kathy walking any distance at all. She advised me her walker was equipped with a seat and, by the way, if I felt I needed to sit down at any time I could use it, too. She offered to push me. Our first belly laugh of the evening!

We dined at The Keg Mansion and decided to review my 'what to say and what not to say' chapter, in case I were to write another book and might want to update any of my suggestions. And, just like that, my suggestions became our suggestions.

I jotted down some of my dear friend's exact words and we reviewed them while I typed our notes back at the Lodge. Kathy wanted to ensure I 'got it right', so after we discussed each thought, I read back what I had written. She seemed to ponder every point for a long time, but I would remind myself this amazing woman had brain cancer and yet she wanted to continue to help others.

The second we arrived back at Kathy's lodging, we took a washroom break before we settled in with our work for the evening.

As Kathy returned to our room, she sat on the side of her bed and, with a big smile on her face, said, "I have just realized something. I'll be dead by the time you finally get this book written, so good luck handling any negative press we receive!"

While that doesn't sound at all funny as I write it years later, I can assure you I took my lead from Kathy and she laughed out loud for the longest time. Her sense of humour was one of the amazing things about her.

Following are our thoughts and suggestions, written in the first person. Sometimes that person is me and other times you're reading Kathy's thoughts.

Let's not exchange stories. Please listen to mine. I wanted to use 'Shut up and listen,' as the lead-in to this point, but Kathy wouldn't have it. "I don't say shut up," she reminded me.

If you come to visit me, and if you ask how I'm doing, I need you to please be quiet and listen to what I have to say. I know you did it differently and you think my treatment should have been like yours and how soon you went back to work and on and on and on. No two cancers are the same and don't get me started on brain cancer compared to your cancer.

Leave your negative energy at home. I'm sorry you've had a bad day, but keep that to yourself until I recover, please and thank you. Quite frankly, I simply can't care about anyone but myself at the moment. Brain cancer is in a whole different world than, say, the non-cancerous mole you had removed from your shoulder.

Kathy asked if she was still in charge of our narrative. I said, "Of course you are. Let me know when you need a break."

"I won't need a break," came her cheeky reply.

Be proactive. If you ask me what you can do to help, please remember I might be too ill to make that decision. So, you could say you were at the grocery store so picked up a few things for my family while you were there. You could suggest you would love to take a turn driving me for treatments or for a doctor's appointment. The list goes on...

Don't be an Internet junkie. If you can't help yourself, then all I ask is that you do not visit me to tell me all about my cancer according to what you found on social media. I'm getting my information from my team and it's hard enough to hear it when they have all the facts, so no Internet diagnoses, please. Carol Ann will be happy to listen to you later...I'll be dead by then, remember?

No belly laugh followed Kathy's comment this time. We don't make fun of having cancer very often, so it's tough to know where our humour will land.

I'll cry if I want to. A cancer survivor will tell you that crying is okay and sometimes it's best to enjoy and share your tears. During our dinner we cried, albeit mainly because there is no washroom on the main floor of the Keg Mansion.

Kathy told our server what she thought of that and then the server reminded us that the Mansion is an historic building and therefore cannot be updated with things like elevators or new plumbing.

I leaned in and whispered to Kathy, "Quick, play the cancer card."

She did not disappoint as she smiled, put her hand over the server's hand and said, "You do know I have brain cancer and at the moment I am living right next door at the Lodge? Meaning, my friend and I need to get out of here so I can go to the bathroom."

Kathy paid our bill and we walked back to the Lodge, where she knew exactly where to locate the washrooms and how to access them.

Once she was comfortably tucked into bed, the laughing and crying began all over again. Memories are made of this.

Every time I've had the pleasure of dining at the Keg Mansion following her death my thoughts are of Kathy. I laugh more than I cry when I share our story now, but the tears are more likely to flow when I'm with close friends who miss Kathy as much as I do.

Say, "I love you," and say it often. Growing up in our home in Wilmot, I rarely heard these three words. This all changed years later, the day my mom was discharged from the hospital following her diagnosis of metastatic breast cancer.

My sisters and I were having dinner with mom around her tiny kitchen table and, as if we did it every day of our lives, we joined hands and all said, *I love you*, first to mom and then to each other. It was a powerful moment for all of us. I will never forget how wonderful it made me feel.

Kathy didn't feel the need to contribute here because, "I say I love you all the time and not only to my family."

I replied with, "Well, I'm happy for you."

Cue the laughter.

Lighten up. Over Billy Minor pie at the Keg Mansion *another* evening, yes, we went a second time and I wasn't even Kathy's 'night nurse,' she shared a funny story about sitting in front of a 'guest' of a cancer patient on the little bus that picked them up daily to take them from the Lodge to the hospital for their treatment.

Kathy sat with her bald head and her gioblastoma tucked away in her brain, while that same 'guest' in the seat directly behind Kathy wouldn't shut up about how short her hairdresser had cut her hair the day before. "I am going to interview a few hairdressers and I might leave my current hairdresser with one less client."

Kathy said she was sorry I wasn't with her on the bus that day because she would have asked me to tell this person to 'shut up' on Kathy's behalf.

At some point Kathy shared this experience with our waiter at the Keg, leading with, "You probably haven't noticed that I'm bald, but how would you feel if you had to listen to this story?"

She had our waiter in tears of laughter before she was half way through the story. I can call that memory up as if it was yesterday, that she was making me laugh out loud over a cancer story.

Play the 'Cancer Card.' When someone begins what you suspect will be a long rant, Kathy and I both want you to know that cancer gives you the permission to interrupt, point both hands at yourself and say, "Hey...cancer here. Let's be quiet for a bit, please."

It works. Trust me, I've been playing the cancer card for over thirty years. Thirty years.

Recognize a good pity-party when you see one, or when you feel one coming on. I still have pity parties!

Kathy loved hearing my pity party stories but had passed away by the time 2021 rolled around. I endured a ten-month-long pity-party when I packed my very loud cough, often called a 'bark', in my suitcase, and headed for Halifax.

Early in 2022, while back in Toronto and under the care of more than a couple of excellent doctors and specialists at Mount Sinai Hospital, I did receive a diagnosis...radiation damage to my left lung + bronchiectasis + a hint of asthma = a chronic lung disease.

Fingers crossed. No pity parties required at the moment. My bark has left the building and I couldn't be more grateful.

Early 2023 I took the Methacholine Asthma Challenge and that's when my diagnosis was updated to include 'a hint' of asthma.

Post-cancer, our 'normal' is not what it once was. I was gutted when a friend said, "Carol Ann, I'm so proud of you. *You act so normal.*"

I had had a mastectomy just a few weeks earlier. This was my normal...my *new normal*. I love this person and if he had only stopped to think what he was about to say before opening his mouth...

Kathy wasn't lucky enough to enjoy a post cancer period in her life. I remind myself of this when I feel a 'whine' of sorts coming on.

Be prepared to lose a friend or two. When my sister's husband, John Dea, was diagnosed with cancer, he fought until his very last breath. He tried with his whole heart to stay with Connie. Following John's death I was stunned to hear comments from Connie's friends.

I was with her and heard a few comments one afternoon as we sat in her Miata, top down, enjoying an ice cream.

"I realize death is hard to deal with but...it was for the best." "You must have known it was coming, kiddo."

I wanted to jump out of the car and give one of the ladies a smack upside the head, but Connie didn't want me to do that. She's kinder that way.

Your thoughts:

42B: Childhood cancer is unforgivable

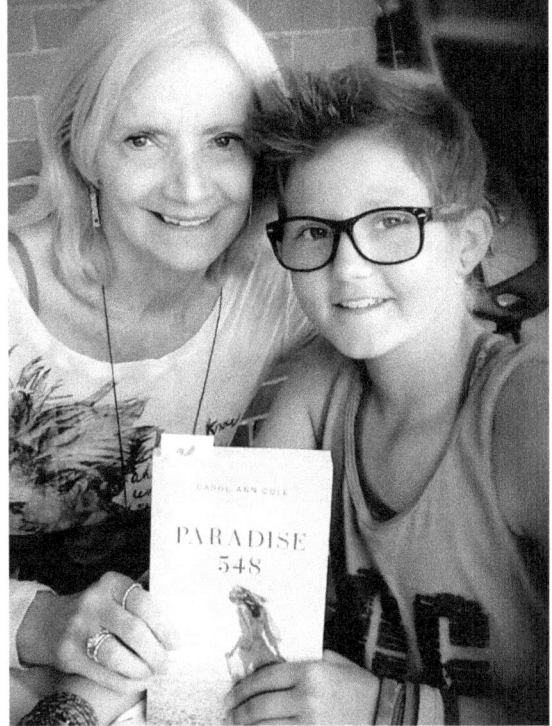

I first reached out to Karissa and her mother because they live near my hometown and I wanted to help. Karissa was eleven years old the first time cancer ravaged her young body. She fought back. I believe she was in remission when I met her on the veranda of my friend Tanya's home. She was proud to be purchasing a copy of my novel with her own money.

These pictures with Karissa are among my most cherished photos.

I asked if it was okay for me to give her a hug. It was.

Not even one year later, the beast came back for Karissa, not realizing she is a warrior and was ready for round two. She fought through a bone marrow transplant while in the Toronto General Hospital. This battle cost Karissa and her mother a repeat of their earlier 150-plus days per year away from home.

Drum roll, please...look at you now, young lady! Cancer-free and with a life to live.

Karissa, I can almost hear you say...

I'm brave.
I'm strong.
I'm intelligent.
I'm silly.
I'm loving.
I'm caring.
I'm beautiful.
I've got the best mom.
I'm invincible.
I'm a warrior.
I'm healthy.
I'm ready.
I win.

And you did!

43: Share with the less-fortunate

We all think differently when it relates to 'our own' money. I understand that.

I'll begin with my own views on tipping. I believe if you decide to leave a tip at a restaurant or elsewhere, you should, if you can, be generous. And tip everyone. I know this one will come back to bite me, because speaking about other people's money is taboo, right? I learned that the hard way many years ago. That's for another day.

A friend of mine shared that in all the years she had worked part-time at Tim Horton's *no one* had ever left a tip on the counter. *OMG, that included me.* I don't know why, but until she raised this with a few of us I had not ever tipped at Tim's.

I changed that immediately and I can proudly tell you that I never leave the counter without putting a bit of money on the counter and saying softly to whoever waited on me, "This is for your tip jar. Thank you." It's always appreciated.

Pay the farmers at the market, at the very least, full value for their work. There is a chance a bit of change might mean more to the vendors than to you. I know many love to barter and I've bartered too when the situation properly presents itself.

It's not only vendors at the market who need our financial assistance. Don't forget the homeless person you see randomly in your 'hood. No need to help every homeless person you meet...pick one.

I'll share a story about my homeless friend. In Halifax in the early 90s I often encountered one particular lady, always in 'her own spot' asking everyone who approached her on Spring Garden Road if they could "Spare any change?"

She would ask once, then her voice would raise if she felt you were about to walk past her. "*Spare. Any. Change?*" If you dared to ignore her a second time she would speak to your back, using some rather vulgar language.

One day, after being the recipient of her foul language, I decided to have a discussion, woman to woman. Some words or names may be changed to not 'out' my friend.

"Hi, there. My name is Carol Ann. May I ask your name, dear?"

"My name is Louise. Can you spare any change? I already asked you twice and I just saw you coming out of the bank."

Ouch! That is aggressive!

Following her comment, Louise spit on her fingers and tried to shape an unruly eyebrow. My heart softened. She knew how she looked.

"I'm not able to spare any change today, but rather than swear at me, if you stop making sure I know every vulgar expression you know, I might be more likely to give you some money." It was early one July when Louise and I had our first encounter.

"If you offer a smile when I see you on the street over the next few months I will have some money for you closer to Christmas. Deal?"

"Yes, and I would really like that." I knew she meant it.

It wasn't long before Louise changed her comments to me as I passed by her corner. Instead of, "Spare any change?" she would say, "It will soon be Christmas," even if Christmas was many months away.

I gave her money in November. I also shared that she was the only person that I was able to help this way, so perhaps we could keep this between us.

"It will be our secret and thank you so much," Louise said. She offered me a big toothless smile and we both moved on.

I watched her to see if she showed any of her street buddies what I had given her. My heart went out to Louise as I watched her cross the street and go straight to an Instabank. I like to think she deposited her Christmas gift.

Several months into the next year, I saw Louise rushing toward me as I turned onto Spring Garden Road from Barrington Street. I was sure she had forgotten our agreement and would be asking me for money.

I was wrong. She was my friend now, and as she approached she again tried to fix up a bit. First the eyebrows, followed by trying to brush away her tears. When she felt she was close enough to yell, her comment broke my heart.

"Miss, my man died. He was very good to me. He always checked on me and sometimes he would buy me a hot dog or something else to eat. I feel so bad…and…and…and I'm so hungry." She opened her arms and gave me a hug. It wasn't uncomfortable at all.

"Louise, I see the hot dog vendor setting up almost in front of us. Let me buy you lunch and you can tell me all about your man."

"This isn't my spot so I have to move. Get me an extra long hot dog and a large order of fries and I'll have whatever you're having to drink." With that she turned and walked away.

I was surprised by her reply but I also understood. Turf was important to my friend.

"It's a date. I will be able to see where your corner is, correct?" I shouted as she moved further and further away from the chip wagon and me. "Is there a chance we can sit down? These high-heeled boots are killing me. Nobody will take your corner, will they?"

I could see she was a bit reluctant as she replied, "Well, I suppose I could sit on one of the benches over there."

"Perfect, but hurry up. There is only one bench left!" I made her smile and I took that as a win.

We sat together, two women who might have started life in similar circumstances. That detail we would never know. Somewhere along the way, Louise fell on hard times. It can happen in a heartbeat.

**There is not much appealing about a broken man or woman.
There is even less appealing about the person
unwilling to lend a hand.**

We can all make a difference in the life of one stranger. One stranger at a time. It's about leaving footprints of kindness wherever you go.

When life blesses you
financially, don't raise
your standard of living.
Raise your standard of
giving.

44: The boy

James and I had been on our own for a number of years and I was wait-ing for the right time to discuss our last name, 'Scott', with him. He was nine at the time and his decision-making skills were well thought out, for the most part, and so I felt he was ready.

On a sunny Sunday morning as we shared windshield time en route to our weekly Dairy Queen visit for our Peanut Buster Parfait I brought it up. "Son, would you mind if I change my name from Scott back to Cole?"

"What? Why?"

"Because I'm a Cole, son. You're a Scott. There would be no change to your name."

"Honestly, mom, I really don't care. Does it affect me at all if I'm not changing my name?"

"I've waited to have this discussion with you, so here we are. If I'm a Cole and you're a Scott would it be embarrassing or awkward for you to explain the difference if anyone asked?"

"I don't think so. Should it?"

"Another example would be each time Bell moves us to another city, and we both know that will happen, as we enrol you for school we might have to explain the difference in our last names to your teachers."

"Think about that, mom. You always seem to know my teachers by their first name anyway. Even the principal, so I can't imagine my name would ever be a problem. As we both know, by the time you talk with my principal I have problems of my own, and they have nothing to do with my last name."

True enough. Funny comments, though. We were both laughing. James was able to laugh at what we will call his decision-making skills at the age of nine.

Part-way through our parfaits I brought us back to our discussion about my name change. "I think we're on the same page, son. We agree that I will change my name to Cole effective with our next move, possibly to Toronto, for our next adventure in a big city."

"Wait! Can I have a couple of things, mom?"

"I'm sure you can. What would you like to have?"

"Think about this." (One of his favourite expressions at that time.) "There wouldn't be any confusion as I get older if I could have my own name in the phone book and in our lobby where they list all the condo owners and how to reach them. If I can have those two things then we have a deal."

"Agreed. I'll attend to those arrangements soon, sir," I said as I reached over to ruffle James' long hair.

We went back to enjoying the silence, but clearly James' young mind was still processing. "As long as I keep my own money invested in our condo, then I'm an owner, right? My name doesn't have to be Cole, right?" He was double-checking the facts and I liked that.

"Your $100.00 investment is safe and sound." Memories are made of this.

Years later, as James married the love of his life, another name change would take place.

Over the years following his wedding, I would learn that being, "Mother of the groom" is not always any easy moniker to wear. I'm sure I'm not alone in this.

I felt lonely, lovely and happy on James' wedding day. I would lose my rank of being first in his heart and I think it's okay to admit that.

Having always hated second place in anything, I would quickly get used to it.

Their son Jalen is now in university and their daughter Lexi is soon to be a teenager. I am firmly in fourth position.

Fourth in my son's heart. Just off the podium!

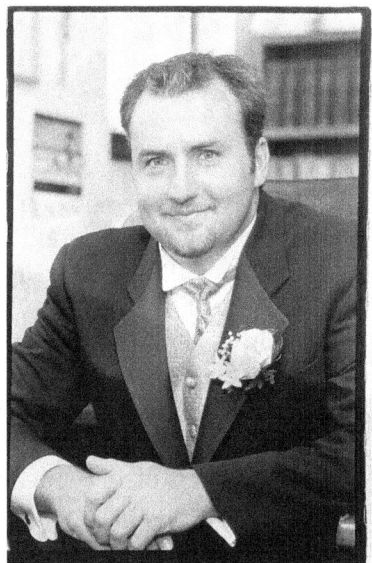

James on his wedding day.

45: Be proud of your hometown

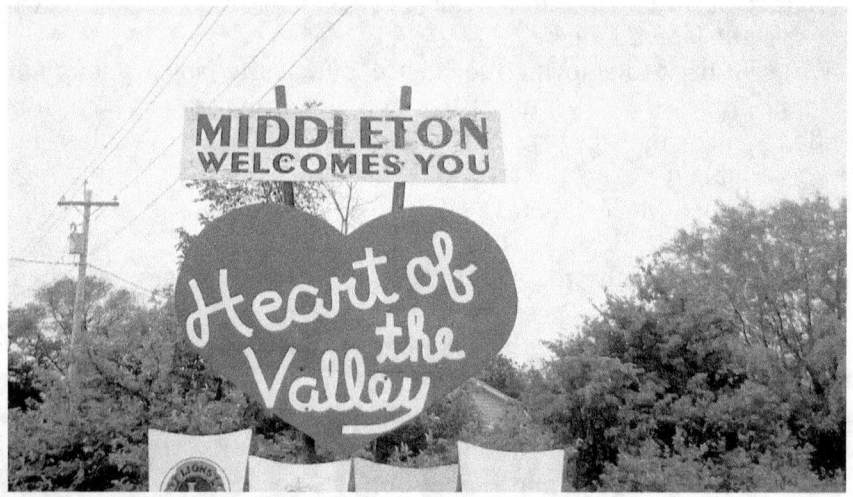

I can hear Bruce Springsteen singing 'My Home Town'.

I have always been proud of where I come from. I grew up in Wilmot, but my roots will forever be in Middleton.

While I was growing up, and in particular when I started going to Middleton Regional High School, I would pass this sign every day.

Grade seven brought with it my first time on a school bus. It would pick me up and drop me off right in front of our house. Five days a week for six years. What could be better than that?

I watched all of my teachers volunteer their time for students who needed extra help. Teachers were often volunteering as they helped each other as well.

I cannot say enough good things about teachers. Did I mention Jalen is going to be a teacher when he graduates from Nipissing University?

Over the years I have volunteered with some wonderful organizations. The Canadian Cancer Society and the Patient Advisory Committee with Mount Sinai Hospital Family Practice in Toronto are two of my current favourites.

I also joined the Middleton Rotary Club. However, for health reasons I was not able to attend weekly meetings and it was difficult to hear some of the voices via Zoom, so I have stepped away for now. I love the Rotary motto and thought I would share it with you. It could be used for everything in life!

Every time you consider doing something or lending your time to a volunteer project in your community consider these four questions:

1. Is it the *truth*?
2. Is it *fair* to all concerned?
3. Will it build *goodwill* and *better friendships*?
4. Will it be *beneficial* to all concerned?

I have to mention a new-to-me restaurant in Middleton at 71 Main Street. 'Angie's Family Restaurant...Nova Scotia Strong.' I mention it for a number of reasons. First, I love the poster on the back wall.

If anything gives us a nudge to eat dessert first, this slogan is it!

To quote, with permission, from Angie's website, "We are a locally owned and operated family restaurant. We offer a comfortable and relaxed dining atmosphere with our menu based around home style comfort food that is sourced locally from our amazing Annapolis Valley."

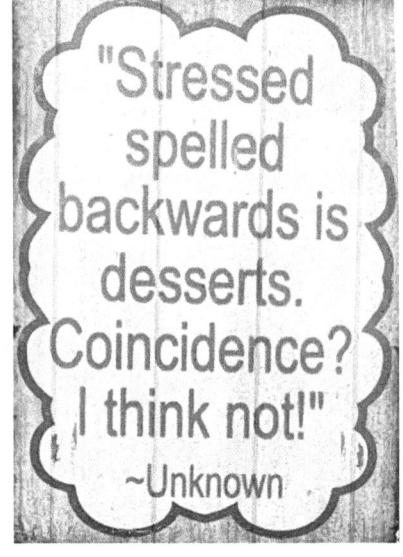

I have yet to order everything on Angie's menu, but if I go back again and again and again I'm sure I will enjoy everything I order. And I will order my dessert first!

46: Mentoring is a gift

My mother was my first mentor, then and always.

Mr. Peppard was my second mentor, then and always.

During the years that I attended Middleton Regional High School, 'Pep' was our physical education teacher. Everyone loved Mr. Peppard, and we still do.

On a personal level, Mr. Peppard knew a bit about my rough and tough relationship with my father...and he understood me. There were days when I felt safer at school.

To this day, he has attended almost every book launch I have had in and around the Middleton/Greenwood area. Mr Peppard seeks me out, gives me a hug, followed by the same question he shares not only with me but with anyone around, "What do I have to buy this time?"

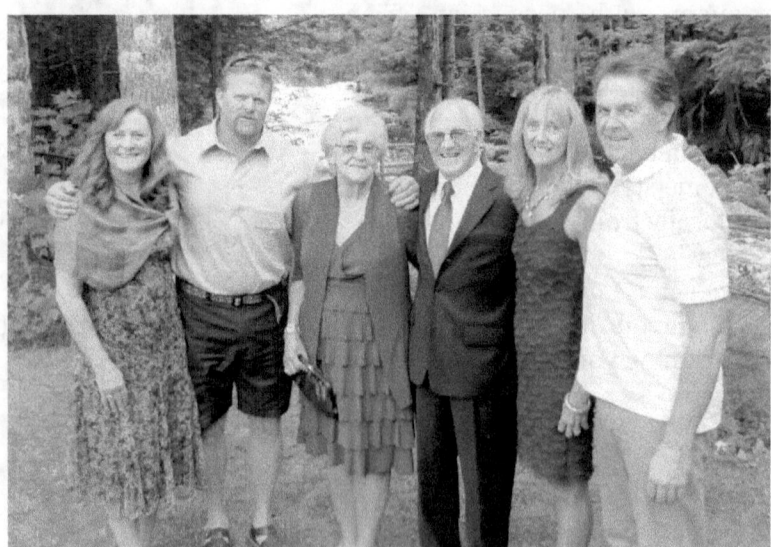

Mr and Mrs Peppard and their four children

I purchased this *TIME* commemorative edition with RBG, as she was known, on the cover. 'A Principled Life 1933-2020.'

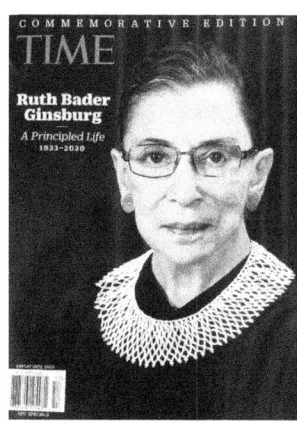

Ruth Bader Ginsburg's accomplishments are extraordinary and I wanted Lexi to have a copy of this issue. If you are unfamiliar with RBG, I encourage you to Google her name. I am looking forward to talking with Lexi about this incredible woman when the time is right. Perhaps once she is in high school. I suspect RBG continues to mentor others from her front-row seat in heaven.

Nelson Mandela...Forgiveness makes you stronger.

I can't say it better than he did, so I am happy to quote Mr. Mandela, who continues to mentor so many years after his death.

I recall a poster in one of the subway cars in Toronto back in the late 70s. I studied it every time I saw it. The poster was of a man obviously just finishing his prison term. He's on the outside of the bars with a few men on the inside looking out. There was a prison in the background just in case the viewer didn't get the message already. The man looked huge in stature and small in confidence.

I will never forget the wording on that poster.

Freedom.
Now the punishment starts.

Before Nelson Mandela left prison he said.

"As I stand before the door to my freedom, I realise that if I do not leave my pain, anger and bitterness behind me, I will still be in prison."

Forgiveness does not make you weak, it sets you free.

Following my second battle with breast cancer in 2008, I wanted to step outside of the cancer arena and volunteer somewhere totally different. I decided to take on a role as 'Writer in Residence' at The Good Neighbours Club on Jarvis Street in Toronto.

The Club is a place where homeless men can go to shower, do their laundry and get a good meal. There is always a lineup when their doors open at 8 am.

The men spend their day at the Club playing pool and various card games, smoking outside, etc. A number of Club members spoke with me about the pride they have when they say, "I spend my days at the Club." So much better than saying they spend their days in a homeless shelter.

Some of the men were skeptical about what I was really doing there. Could I be a nurse and, if so, could I take a look at something? Or maybe a lawyer there to give advice? Even though there were posters put up throughout the Club introducing me as a writer offering to help them write a letter home, or journal their life from Bay Street to homelessness. I was there every Wednesday from 10 am until 12.

Being homeless or incarcerated humbled some, not all, of these men.

For my first session I brought my laptop along, thinking I could type a letter, print it right there and hand it over to the Club member who had dictated his letter to me. For the most part, my laptop was not 'trusted.' How could they trust me to not have already sent their letter to someone without their permission? Lesson learned, I bought only pen and paper for the rest of my gig.

I was not only a writer while there. I provided a listening ear, a human who would sit and talk with them, maybe open a few doors if someone, for example, could not afford a bus pass.

My son was not totally supportive of me in this volunteer position. He worried that someone might frighten me or, worse, physically hurt me. I promised James I would walk away the day that happened.

And I did.

47: Working together works

Working together has always been important to me, regardless of who might rank highest on the company payroll. Starting with my first job as a stenographer with the Bank of Nova Scotia and then with Bell, when asked what my job included I have always replied with a hint of humour, "Oh, I have a big job at the Bell." I played for all the marbles so every job was a big job. With my chosen response to every query about my job I like to think I cut the, "Atta-girl" comments in half.

Additionally, this all but eliminated the over-used line from men (think mid 60s), "I hear you're a typist at Bell. Bell is always going to need a typist or two, so *good for you, young lady*...you have a job for life."

Following are examples of words that speak to inclusivity...and re-member, always try to call your teammates by name.

> 'Ken and I are on the same team.'
> 'Bill and I work well together.'
> 'Barb and I started working here on the same day.'
> 'Nik is new to our country and I have promised him we are a team that strives for inclusiveness in everything we do. He's anxious to get to know all of you.'

'Buddy works for me,' is an example of an old-school boss needing every-one to know who the boss is and that everyone else works under him. Give it a bit more time; this attitude is almost a thing of the past.

**Allow your team to work *with* you, not *for* you.
And, if you can, call them by name.**

Your thoughts:

Part 2:

Poetry & song and

keeping it all in one place

I am happy to share several stanzas from a few of my favourite poems and songs. I'm curious to know if the messages 'speak' to you as they have to me over the years. I read each poem differently at my current age than I might have years ago but they all remain important to me.

48: Cat's in the Cradle

My son was just starting school when this song was released, so while he heard me singing it over and over he didn't connect the dots until he was a few years older. During my Bell career, my son knew I worked late almost every day and again on the weekend. (I'm not proud of that, just for the record. It's simply a fact.)

'Cat's in the Cradle' is a song that says it all. It describes me. Harry Chapin found the poem his wife had written and tucked away in a dresser drawer. Harry sat down and wrote the music. The rest, as they say, is history.

James and I continue to sing 'Cat's in the Cradle' when it seems one of us is, in the opinion of the other, just a bit too busy. I am including only the words closer to the end of the song, (with an apology for changing the parent from male to female.)

> ...I've long since retired,
> My son has moved away,
> I called him up just the other day.
> I said, "I'd like to see you if you don't mind."
> He said, "I'd love to, mom, if I can find the time
> You see, my new job's a hassle, and the kids have the flu,
> But it's sure nice talking to you, mom
> It's been sure nice talking to you."
> As I hung up the phone, it occurred to me
> He'd grown up just like me
> My boy was just like me.
>
> Harry Chapin, 1974

In 1982, James was turning thirteen and we had just been transferred to Montreal. I thought a portrait was in order...albeit I'm not quite sure why

I made the decision that we should wear matching burgundy turtleneck sweaters.

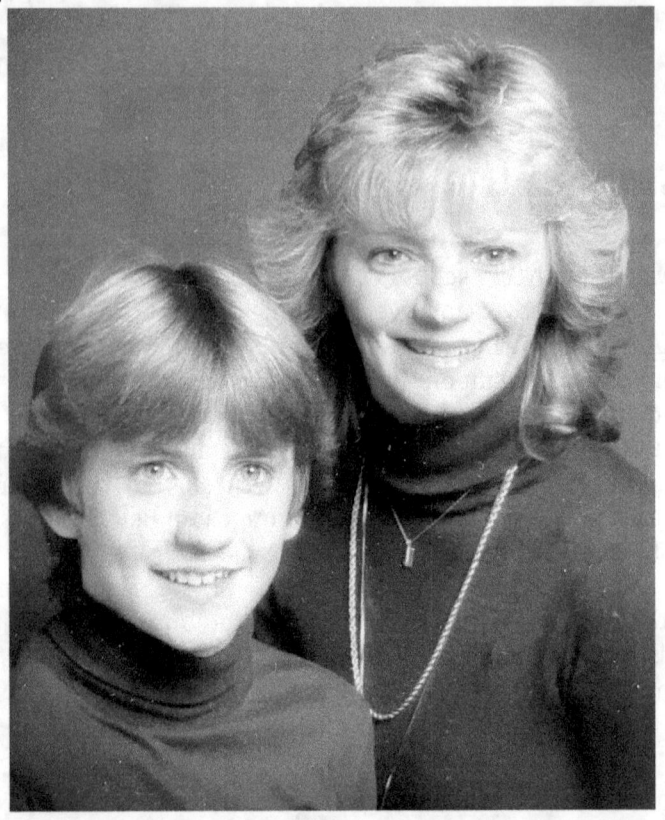

When I had the photo enlarged to sit on my office desk at 1050 Beaver Hall Hill in downtown Montreal, I took a fair bit of ribbing from the men, in particular.

"Why does your kid have to dress the same as you?"

"Oh, your poor kid. Does he have to wear matchy-matchy every day?"

The only comment that bothered me is one I will never forget. Partly because it was true that I spent too many hours at the office. Comments like this were thrown around in late 70s and 80s when many men felt women who wanted to climb the corporate ladder were taking promotions away from them and felt that they were more deserving of the job. "Exactly who is raising your kid while you are non-stop-working at the office?"

Ouch.

49: Slow dance

This poem reminds us that when we tell a child we're "busy right now", we often fail to see the sadness reflected in his or her face. We hurry up so we can slow down. I've been there.

I contacted David L. Weatherford in the early 90s to request permission to share his poem 'Slow Dance' in my professional speaking life as well as in print. He was very gracious and his permission continues to be much appreciated.

Slow Dance

Have you ever watched kids on a merry-go-round?
Or listened to rain slapping the ground?

Ever followed a butterfly's erratic flight?
Or gazed at the sun fading into the night?

You better slow down.

Don't dance so fast.
Time is short.

The music won't last.

Do you run through each day on the fly?
When you ask, "How are you?" do you hear the reply?

When the day is done, do you lie in your bed,
with the next hundred chores, running through your head?

Ever told your child, we'll do it tomorrow,

and in your haste, not see his sorrow?

Ever lost touch, let a good friendship die,
'cause you never had time to call and say hi?

You better slow down.

Don't dance so fast.

Time is short.

The music won't last.

When you run so fast to get somewhere
you miss half the fun of getting there.

When you worry and hurry through your day,
It's like an unopened gift, thrown away.

Life is not a race,

So take it slower.
Hear the music

before the song is over.

David is a child psychologist with published poems in *Chicken Soup for the Soul.* If you want to enjoy more of his beautiful writings, please visit davidlweatherford.com.

Only in my post-Bell careers and in retirement have I learned to slow dance rather than running through each day. This poem doesn't just speak to me. It screams at me!

50: The dash

In the mid 90s Tracey shared this poem with me, and in turn I have shared 'The Dash' with thousands of individuals over the years.

This poem is about how we spend *our* dash that will appear on our grave marker between the date of our birth and the day we die. It speaks to how we might spend our dash every day. Each day arrives with a blank page, a new dash...ready for you to create memories as you decide how you want to spend your day.

Many years ago, I contacted the author of 'The Dash', Linda Ellis, to seek permission to share her poem. We agreed on an honorarium and I sent a check immediately.

I touched base with her again while writing this book. I am proud to say I consider Linda a friend.

Her poem contains nine stanzas in total. I encourage you to look it up. Linda has sold the rights to her poem and I hesitate to upset anyone, so I have not included the full poem here. It's easy to find on the Internet if you're interested. If you can't find it, I can send it to you.

The Dash

I read of a man
who stood to speak
at the funeral of a friend.
He referred to the dates
on her tombstone
from the beginning...
to the end.
...
It matters not how much we own
The cars. The House. The cash.

Learning to Slow Dance

What matters is how we live and love
And how we spend our dash.
...
So, when your eulogy is being read
with your life's actions to rehash
would you be proud
of the things they say
about how you spend your dash?

Linda Ellis

51: No title at all

The next poem I have chosen to share with you has no title at all.

I have researched this omission and I believe the author, Mother Teresa, made a conscious decision to allow everyone who read her beautiful poem to give it their own title. Even without a title, these words speak volumes.

If you're a parent, read this poem with your child in mind. It will make you think.

And, if you're not a parent, read it with a special someone in mind. Maybe someone you helped many years ago and they feel like family to you today.

> You will teach them to fly, but they will not fly your flight.
> You will teach them to dream, but they will not dream your dream.
> You will teach them to live, but they will not live your life.
> Nevertheless, in every flight, in every life, in every dream,
> the print of the
> way you taught them will remain.
>
> from *Be Like Francis*

I would love it if we could get this poem in the hands of every parent we know. As a mother and a nana I can relate. Can you?

Jot your thoughts here for those who, one day, you will leave behind. Memories are made of this.

52: All I really need to know I learned in kindergarten

Here is the 'Storyteller's Creed', as quoted in several of Robert Fulghum's books:

> I believe that imagination is stronger than knowledge. That myth is more potent than history. That dreams are more powerful than facts. That hope always triumphs over experience. That laughter is the only cure for grief. And I believe that love is stronger than death.

I am only sharing a portion of his poem with you, but I think it will explain why I kept a huge framed copy of this poem on my many different office walls throughout my career.

All I really need to know I learned in kindergarten speaks to me.

One of the numerous talks I have given through the years is called 'Five Things You Should Do Every Single Day.' My talking notes consisted of five words:

> Listen
> Learn
> Look
> Share
> Care

Each word came with a personal story, from my heart. My stories were based on Robert Fulghum's poem and some of his additional writings.

All I really need to know I learned in kindergarten (excerpt)

Most of what I really need
To know about how to live
And what to do and how to be
I learned in kindergarten...
These are the things I learned:
Share everything.

Play fair.
Don't hit people.
Put things back where you found them.
Clean up your own mess.
Live a balanced life –

Robert Fulghum

Your thoughts:

Part 3:

Family and friends

This section is different in format.
I have turned it over to family members and friends.
A few contributors are septuagenarians...only a few!

53: From my friend Sherilyn M Fritz

Love unconditionally

It is important to love others as they are and not as what we expect them to be.

I had to learn this with my children as they were growing up, and I'm proud to share this in Carol Ann's book. I want to remind everyone how important acceptance is.

[Carol Ann whispers: In late September 2023 I had the pleasure of talking with Sherilyn at the Middleton Library where I was launching my fifth book in The Paradise Series. I was so happy to see Sherilyn walk through the door. We had a lovely visit and she encouraged all who were there that day to discuss acceptance with their family and ensure that we love others as they are and without judgment.]

54: Donna Sabean

Donna Sabean is my cousin. I knew her in our youth as Madonna Cole. As often happens, we grow up, we move in different directions and years rush by.

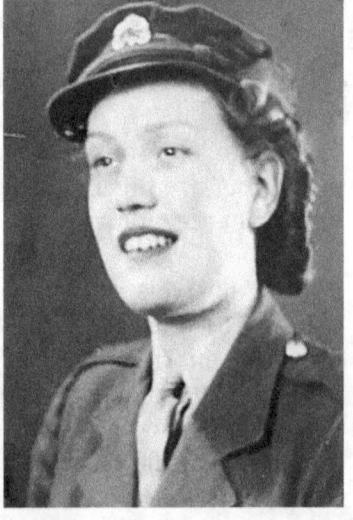

Today, we live in the same province, for the most part, and see each other as often as we can. I enjoy spending time with Donna and her husband, Joey. Additionally, Donna is a great cook, which makes visiting their home even more inviting!

Donna's mother, Joyce Cole, was from the UK and spoke with a proper English accent. (My mother was from the Acadian South Shore in Nova Scotia and spoke with her Acadian-French accent.)

Joyce also served her country. War broke out in 1939 when she was seventeen. At twenty-one she enlisted in the army and served in the Royal Canadian Corps of Signals (RCCS.) The RCCS was responsible for land communication and signalling. When the Canadian Army, Royal Canadian Air Force and Royal Canadian Navy were unified in 1968 to form the Canadian Forces, the RCCS was amalgamated into the Canadian Forces' Communications and Electronic Branch.

On May 9th, 1945, Joyce was discharged.

Married to Ross Cole, Joyce came to Canada as a war bride, landing at Pier 21 in Halifax in 1945. Mother to five children, Joyce had a busy life in Canada, settling in the Annapolis Valley in Nova Scotia. She passed away in 1998.

To me this intelligent and beautiful lady was 'Auntie Joyce.'

Poetry is one way my cousin expresses herself, and while I have read dozens and dozens of Donna's poems. One in particular speaks to me.

My Mom

You took my Mom too soon Lord, I miss her very much.
I wish you could send her back, so I could feel her tender touch.

I miss her funny laughter and the way that she would speak.
With that polished English accent not all of us could speak.

I miss her every day, but I feel her in my heart.
I wish that we could find a way to go back to the start.

Mom didn't always have the life that she deserved to have.
She had a lot of trouble with my dad.

She could make a dollar stretch to include many things
as she struggled each day to give us everything.

We laughed and we cried together as she became so very ill.
But she never once complained ...she was never one to quit.

And when her time drew near Lord, we never left her side.
I held her hand as she died.

I love my mom so dearly Lord, and I miss her every day.
If she was with me today I know what I would say.

"Thank you very much Mom, you did your very best."
I know now, that my mother deserves this nice long rest.

Please keep Mom in your grace Lord, and surround her with your love.
Remind her we will meet again when you take me up above.

I hope to be as faithful as I knew my Mom to be.
When I look to heaven Lord, I know that's where she will be.

Madonna Sabean 2013

55: Lorraine Rosenal

My sister Lorraine, and I are middle-sisters, with Lois and Connie on either side of us.

Lorraine's words offer food for thought when forming friendships. Some friendships endure the test of time. Some do not.

Hi Carol Ann

I'm thinking about your request for truths we've learned as we age.

The one that comes to mind is that when I've picked my friends well, I can have faith that they will be with me through thick and thin. And when family is at a distance, friends are often the first to provide support.

Life would be even harder without friends.

Love,
Lorraine

56: Ron Bryant

Ron is a friend from our Bell days together.

Appreciate what you have while you still have it.
Say the things now that you probably will later wish you had said.

> Sometimes
> it's not the song
> that makes
> you emotional.
> It's the people,
> and the things
> that come to your mind
> when you hear it.

57: Peter Booth and his Mum-pride

Peter and I were on the same Bell team many years ago. One day it fell to me to make the drive to Peterborough to deliver bad news to Peter and his teammates. We were shutting their department down.

It was an ugly exchange.

I believed then and I believe now that bad news, especially bad news, should be delivered face to face. I wasn't expecting the shellacking that came my way and I wore it for several days. It was still the right thing to do.

Many years later I ran into Peter and his peers at a Bell Pensioners meeting. I saw him walking towards me and I swear I could tell he had mellowed (thank God). Peter quietly shared a personal story involving his wife, Carol.

In that moment, something shifted between us. I believe we both decided to seize the moment. Life is short.

We now keep in touch and I'm proud to say both Pete and Carol are friends of mine.

Following is Peter's story.

Hi, Carol Ann,

I hit seventy-five in 2021. I'm officially an old guy and this is an old-guy snow-shovelling story.

Carol makes some grand meals. One day she cooked a turkey, complete with dressing, potatoes, carrots, turnip, parsnips and gravy. Just grand, and the next day we had turkey sandwiches.

Can't have turkey sandwiches without really fresh bread. I got in my truck and drove down to Wild Flower Bakery for a loaf of white bread. Ended up with my loaf of bread, four huge, warm croissants, and the last blueberry pie.

Now, I know what you're thinking...none of this has anything to do with snow and my Mum-pride.

I'm a little out of chronological order, but that's just me. I returned home from the bakery with the use of my four-wheel drive. Immediately, I had a warm croissant with lots of butter. Took one into mum and she did the same.

I had to bring in my air hose and compressor...another story for another time.

Now I'll go back to my story about being seventy-five and shovelling snow. It had to be done so I go outside again and start shovelling the front deck. Those who have been here know that I don't do a great job but it's serviceable...front deck and maybe four feet in from the driveway.

I grab my shovel and head around to the west side of the house, to the gate to mum's patio. Mum has a walled-in patio maybe twenty-five feet square. There are two paths to shovel, maybe a total of thirty feet plus a little path to a hole in the wall so mum's feral cat, Klutie, can come in for her feed without having to challenge the pool area and get past Molly.

Finally, here comes Pete carrying his shovel and ready to clear the path, but guess what? It's already shovelled. I guess I'm not quick enough for this tenant. So, I started shovelling and suddenly the apartment door opens.

Mum comes outside. "Oh, Peter, please be careful. The snow is so heavy and it's dangerous for you. I was going to finish that later."

So there you have it...a snow-shovelling story about me at seventy-five years of age, and my Mum, who turned 98 years young in June of 2023. To this day, she is still watching out for me.

"Oh, Peter, please be careful."

My mum is absolutely awesome.

58: Tom DeYoung

Tom is one of my Halifax-based friends.
I first met him and his wife, Rita, when I moved to a condo in Halifax during the late 90s.
We have kept in touch. The following is from Tom. (Rita passed away in late 2021. Again Tom, I'm so sorry for your loss.)

Hi, Carol Ann,

My dad passed away when I was six, so our mom raised my sister and me. I am now over eighty years old...so here goes.

First on my list of what I would say to the younger generation would be to stay in school and get a good education. I know it sounds like a standard 'line', but I believe, more than ever, that the best jobs go to the people with the most education. You can chase your dreams and complete your education, too. Stay in school. Please.

I quit school half-way through grade nine. My averages were seventy-five or more, but I was not a school person. I tried different jobs and finally went to trade school. One of the things I have learned is that you always learn something that you can use down the road.

My children, Laura and Richard, both finished high school. My son has been working for the Marriott for over twenty-five years. My daughter went to what was called, at the time, Miss Murphy's Business College, where she completed a secretarial course. After various jobs she became executive assistant for two national not-for-profit organizations.

Laura accepted the position of secretary to the CEO of The National Gallery of Canada Foundation. Her office is in her home. She can stay right here in Nova Scotia! I say that's even better than the promotion. I am proud of both Laura and Richard for all they have achieved and for the adults they have become.

Life's Lessons for me include…

Family comes first, always.
Take each day as it comes. Yesterday is behind you and tomorrow hasn't arrived.
Ask questions about your family. I didn't and am sorry for it.
Be proud of your children and grandkids. I am so proud of mine.
Be grateful for your health. Never take it for granted.
Never stop reading and learning.
Never trust a politician.
Be grateful for your friends. You might need them in the future.

Would I have done things differently if I had stayed in school? Who knows?

When you retire, you should have a plan to keep yourself busy.

Finally, and perhaps my most important message to pass on, is something I worry about. This might be my only worry.

What kind of world are we leaving for our grandkids?

Thanks for asking me to contribute, Carol Ann. I really appreciate it.

Tom

59: Bill Valcour

Bill I and worked together for a number of years during our careers with Bell Canada. He is intelligent, motivated, detail-oriented, caring, loyal, has a wicked sense of humour and is a good friend of mine.

As you read Bill's story, do me a favour and stick with it until he gets to life after career, because that is where you will see the real Bill Valcour, as I know him today.

Hi, Carol Ann,

The acquisition of knowledge or skills through experience, study, or by being taught is the meaning of learnings.

At mid-century I was confident and comfortable in life, perhaps leaning towards arrogance, although I didn't see the latter at the time.

My eldest son returned home in a wheelchair to live with Linda and me, as the result of a horrendous industrial accident. When he was mostly recovered he once again moved out on his own.

I could write a book on learnings during the period of time. I love him but was pleased he was leaving.

My youngest son, in his third decade of life, had earned another degree and was finally entering the workforce, albeit thousands of miles away. The arrogance and pride shows here. At times, I refer to him as my son, the Doctor.

In over three decades employed by the same company, I was confident in my job. I wanted to be part of the solution, not shown the door. My career was evolving and I was open to change.

Then it happened. I received a phone call from a headhunter.

I was on an airplane and behind a desk overseas in less than two days, with that nagging uneasy and uncomfortable feeling.

I was only home one weekend out of six. Prior to taking this position, my spouse and I had never lived apart. I would arrive home after six weeks, a bouquet of flowers in one hand and luggage in the other, the lights were all on, a pet peeve of mine, but nobody was home. We were living separate lives.

I was just learning how important my family was, and is, to me.

I was approaching the second year overseas when another head-hunter contacted me. Could I now become a bragger?

The offer was attractive, in Canada, executive position (Vice President). I made a hasty exit for the airport. Family life was restored.

I did seek out alternate employment, around the same money but bolstering my sometimes-showing arrogance. Now I was President. I like this word following my name. Approaching the two-year anniversary, it was the right time to sell.

I still do some consulting. Albeit in the mid septuagenarian timeline of my life I do have a long-overdue retirement plan. I have promised my spouse I will retire upon reaching octogenarian status.

I count my blessings daily. I admit some of the blessings are material-istic, including my Florida home.

That's where I was when a call came from home. My sister was ill and could no longer care for mother. I returned home. Three months later my sister had died, and all that time my spouse and I had been living apart... she in the sun and me in the cold homeland.

My mother's name had been on the Long Term Care Home list for over a year. Moving my mother to the Home was the most difficult thing I had ever done in my entire life. I think of that often. The Home had a profes-sional appearance and I was pleased the room was private. I equipped my mother's room with a large screen television, power recliner, and private phone line.

While the Home had a professional appearance, the care it provided bordered on criminal. Every day brought a new crisis. I would visit every day and, upon arrival, it was like I was the bad smell. Everyone ran from me.

After a few months, the situation calmed to almost acceptable and I left for a two-week vacation in Florida. The day I arrived a phone call from the Home advised that my mother had been moved to the hospital.

I returned immediately and arrived one day before her passing.

The revelations of life in Long Term Care homes during the pandemic absolutely destroyed me. I don't talk about it, but through uncaring and neglect the Home killed my mother.

While still grieving my mother and sister, I welcomed a calming period in my life. Or, so I thought.

My youngest son, the Doctor, over a period of eighteen months, was diagnosed with two different types of cancer, resulting in three surgeries. The survival rates on both cancers were a concern. A number of years have passed and he is recovered and cancer-free. While this is a relief, I remain guarded.

During my son's recovery, I was diagnosed with cancer myself, a type that has a high survival rate but was shocking all the same.

The diagnosis was double-checked and the process was quick, a surgery and a return to normal life...again, so I thought.

A culmination of the above experiences took a toll on my emotional well-being. I had always been strong...not any longer. I have been reduced to an emotional wreck. I lose my composure during some television commercials, never mind the news or a sad movie. I have sought counselling and it helped, perhaps not with the emotions but with the reaction and control.

My spouse has had a heart condition for years, treated with medication, and recently deteriorated to the point that she required surgery. In the range of heart surgeries it was a minor procedure but still of concern.

During the COVID pandemic the surgery was scheduled and I watched my wife walk away from me and into the hospital for heart surgery without me: pandemic protocols kept me out.

I was overwhelmed...it was an epiphany. Family is all that matters.

I drove home for the wait. The call came...all was okay.

A couple of weeks after returning home she experienced severe arrhythmia difficulty. Paramedics were summoned. By the time they arrived, all had calmed and returned to normal. But while she was still connected to the heart monitor, her heart suddenly stopped.

It was a total panic for a few moments until her heart restarted...back to the hospital.

As of writing this, life is calm; my spouse has returned home, a few minor arrhythmia episodes and I have reasonable control of my emotions. It is surprising and perhaps disappointing that it took family deaths and life-threatening illnesses in the family to bring a full realization of the love and appreciation I have of my family.

As I write this we are still suffering from the aftereffects of a worldwide pandemic.

I remain a candidate for Compliance Poster Boy.

All part of the new me.

60: Rob Koldenhof

I met Rob in 1981, when I transferred to Bell's Installation and Repair department. We were part of the Rouge River District team. Rob ensures we keep in touch. I consider Rob and his wife, Rose, friends of mine.

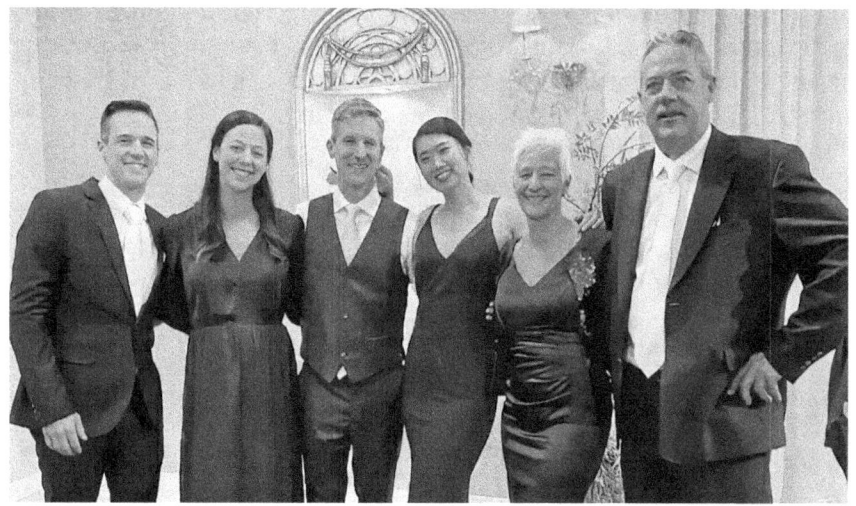

Rob and Rose, with their three children, plus their daughter-in-law!

The COVID virus hit me harder than SARS had years ago. Perhaps 'harder' isn't the right word. It caused me more concern probably because of my age, sixty-four at the time.

At the onset of COVID, Rose and I were returning from our annual two-week getaway in Cancun, Mexico. We got back early in March, 2020.

Shortly thereafter, when no one really knew much about this virus, other than that it was spreading quickly and uncontrollably, I took five months off from my part-time job at NAPA, the National Automotive Parts Association, which was considered an essential service.

I was able to keep myself occupied, for the most part.

I attempted to learn Michael Jackson's 'Moonwalk.' Lacking the speed, balance and foot-coordination required, I was unsuccessful.

I learned how to do some basic sewing using a sewing machine. And I baked white crusty bread. Who didn't bake a loaf during COVID? And if you didn't, you knew someone who did.

One thing I decided to do was reach out and have phone conversations with colleagues from my past at Bell. Every one of those conversations has been rewarding and uplifting. In each case it appeared the recipient was also appreciative of the call. I will continue to reach out long after COVID subsides.

Texting and email have their place in society and are, of course, legitimate forms of communication. But a phone call allows you to hear the laughter, enjoy the banter, and listen to the vocal inflections as the conversation continues. Nothing like a phone call to a person from your past, yet far from the physical conversations, which I miss more than I had realized. I'll be calling you, CA...you're on my list.

Our three kids all moved out many years ago. The oldest turned 40 in 2022, resides in Calgary and is working for Telus. The second son has been in Japan, working as an English language teacher for the last twelve or thirteen years. Our third child resides in Bowmanville, ON with her husband and their two young children. Rose and I have learned that being grandparents is sweet.

We've not been all together since sometime around 2010. In October, 2021, our son in Japan announced his plans to marry his Japanese sweetheart in November of 2022. Going to Japan had never been on our bucket list, but that changed.

As we planned and booked our travel for the event, the universe opened doors as it always does.

This trek around a large portion of the planet was scheduled to begin in October 2022. Our journey would take us from London, ON to Kelowna, BC, where I currently have a younger sister and her family. Another sibling has plans to move to BC from Brampton, ON in 2022. We're hoping a third sibling living in Edmonton, AB will join us for a "Christmas in October."

As a result of the wedding in Japan, our son from Calgary and our daughter in Bowmanville will also be joining us for the celebration. Two family reunions over the course of three weeks, one of which is fourteen hours away and in a location none of us ever dreamed we might visit. Life is pretty spectacular.

Having said all that, I know how blessed we are while others are struggling. Looking beyond Canada, proper medical assistance doesn't exist for those living in poorer countries, refugee camps, in tents, etc. Most have little food or water. To add COVID to their world seemed cruel.

I try to think of these individuals, especially when I complain that the golf courses are closed once again, or that I'm in a 50+ person lineup outside of my closest COSTCO.

I need to do better, even after COVID. I need to think of the people in the camps and the poorer countries more often than I do. I am a very fortunate individual and thankful for all that I have.

All in all, I'm improving as a person and that's a good thing. Cheers!

On a personal level, CAC, this book is a great idea. Thanks for writing it and thanks for reaching out to some of us for our input.

Rob and Rose

Distance doesn't separate people, silence does.

61: In memory of Bill Egan

Bill Egan belonged. Wherever he went, he belonged.

The final flurry of e-mails I exchanged with Bill was during his last few months alive. Bill knew his time was limited, but he was still hoping for an-other five years. He needed a miracle, yet he was positive and happy in the moment.

Bill asked if I had any advice he could take away with him. I encouraged him to say, "I love you," to everyone and Bill quickly interrupted to say, "Hell, I say that to everybody, so I've got that covered."

We talked about 'when it's time' and did I think he would know. All I could say was that everyone handles this differently, and when the time came for him to rest, his family would understand.

Bill, always with humour, asked if 'dancing on his grave' would be frowned on. I suggested we would dance all around his grave.

Just as I was about to hang up came one more smile from a man who, for five whole years, battled this beast we call cancer.

"Hey, let's meet up at the next Bell hockey tournament. And don't forget, you owe me a beer. Make that two!"

The following is with permission of Bill's family.

OBITUARY
William "Bill" Joseph Egan
AUGUST 27, 1954 – APRIL 11, 2021

It is with the heaviest heart that we announce the passing of William (Bill or Billy) Joseph Egan on April 11, 2021 at the age of 66 years. Bill fiercely battled cancer for five years, constantly impressing us all with his strength, undergoing chemotherapy for the duration.

Bill loved blaring loud music at the cottage and dancing all night long. He taught us to take pride in whatever work we did...he worked in the telecommunications industry for over 40 years. He was one of the most selfless humans you can imagine and would do anything for his family.

We are happy that your suffering is finally over. We know you were going through all of it for us.

Our sincerest thanks to Dr. Chan, and the care workers of Lakeridge Health.

Dad, we are sure you are up there with your Mum, Dad, Matt and Bob, causing trouble and looking down on us with love.

Rest in Peace, Papa Bill❤

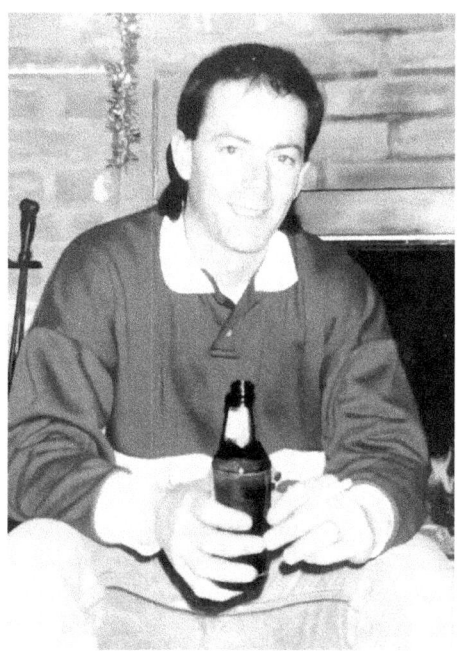

62: Faith Deloughery

Faith and I have been friends for many years. Her kindness, love for others and joy in being able to treat others with kindness is infectious. In her words...

Kindness is simply empathy and generosity: sharing your time, your money, treating others to a bit of yourself. For me, it's gift-giving, over-tipping, trying to stay aware of what people might need and how can I be of service, wanting to bring joy to others.

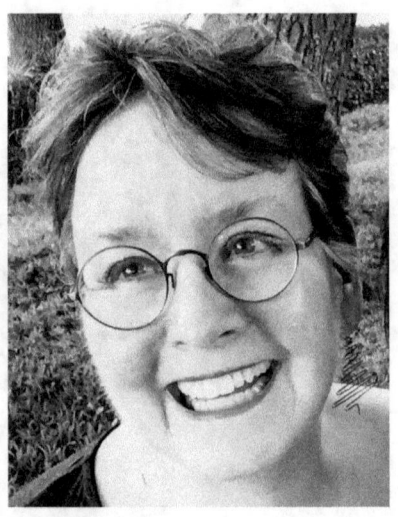

Today it has become a richer and more fulfilling experience for me.

It is my wish that my kind gestures inspire others to pass it on. Let that be my legacy.

As Maya Angelou reminds us, "Your legacy is every life that you touch."

With love,
Faith

63: Life can change in a minute

I have kept the poem that follows for this chapter for a reason.

Early in my professional speaking career I shared "Around the Corner" with an audience, not to silence them but to encourage everyone to call that friend or that special someone now...not later. Talk about falling flat in front of a sizable audience. I had forgotten to set up the true meaning of the poem. The silence was defeating. Lesson Learned.

I recovered, somewhat, and I did share this poem some time later with audience members, but this time I set the stage prior to reading it. I shared my experience of the uncomfortable silence that resonates from an audience and that only the speaker can hear, and how frightened I was for that second when I tried to figure out if 'coming back' from this silence was even possible.

Around the Corner

Around the corner I have a friend,
In this great city that has no end.
Yet days go by and weeks rush on,
And before I know it, a year has gone.
And I never see my old friend's face,
For life is a swift and terrible race.
He knows I like him just as well,
As in days when I rang his bell.
And he rang mine.
But we were younger then,
And now we are busy, tired men.
Tired of playing a foolish game.
Tired of trying to make a name.

"Tomorrow" I say!
"I will call on Jim.
Just to show,
That I'm thinking of him."
But, tomorrow comes and tomorrow goes,
And, distance between us grows and grows.

Around the corner, yet miles away,
"Here's a telegram sir.
Jim died today."
And that's what we get and deserve in the end,
Around the corner, a vanished friend.

Charles Hanson Towne (1877–1949)

At this chapter in my life, I, like you, have lost friends, work colleagues, and family members. It's the circle of life, yet that doesn't make it any easier to hear of a friend's death.

Never leave it until tomorrow to make that call. Never.

If you're putting that call off because you don't know what to say, say that. 'I'm struggling to find the right words and I don't want to upset you by saying the wrong thing,' is better than saying nothing. If you are reluctant to do this, I ask you to please try it...just once. You will see that it helps the person you are struggling to speak with a million times more than it helps you.

During and following COVID I have witnessed a rejuvenated kindness, with both women and men showing kindness towards others. We reach out more often...we actually call each other on the phone. We care.

Women have always, or almost always, shown emotion, but now I see men letting their emotions out and not even apologizing for it. Never apologize for tears.

If reading this chapter has left you feeling down, that was not my intent. The fact is, we think we have time, but we often do not. Make that call.

To end this chapter with a total change of topic and a lighter footprint of kindness...

When I fell, June 2023, after friends and family got caught up on, "What happened?" the talk often turned to my shoe collection. In particular my high-heeled shoes. "Surely to God you won't ever wear those again?"

My response to date has been to agree to dispose of my 'killer' high-heeled shoes in one way or another. I have given some away to someone who will use them and love them, I have decorated corners of my home with some and, yes, I have put several pairs in the garbage. I'm learning as I go.

Currently I am looking for a pair of red boots with a much lower heel to replace my entire collection to date. It's not an easy assignment.

„If someone tells you that you
have enough shoes,
stop talking to them.
You don´t need that kind of
negativity in your life."

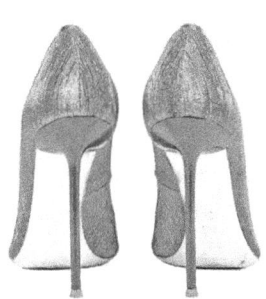

64: Kindness, Comfort Hearts, and cancer

I believe we can find ways to be helpful to others every day. Every morning that we leave our home to face the world, we need to be humble. Love from your heart, say it out loud, listen with both ears and be ready to extend your hand to others. Be grateful.

> A person's most
> useful asset is
> not a head full of
> knowledge, but a
> heart full of love
> an ear ready to listen
> and
> a hand willing to help.

I am extremely proud to be the founder of The Comfort Heart Initiative in memory of my mom, pictured at right, Mary Rose Cole (d'Entremont).

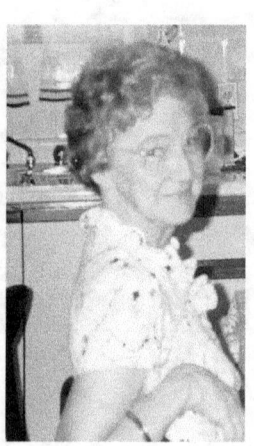

While I was home on vacation in 1995ish, a sign caught my eye...Ocean Art Pewter... a beautiful, welcoming, artsy store near Prospect, NS.

It wasn't until I was paying for gifts I had purchased that a small wicker basket caught my eye. A red-and-white-checkered napkin was spread out proudly in the wicker basket to display 'Worry Hearts.' The tiny pewter heart came with a small card that read...

**Worry night
Worry day
Wish all your
Worries away.**

Over the next year Worry Hearts became Comfort Hearts and the rest, as they say, is history. Every Comfort Heart sold is in memory of my mother.

May Ocean, founder and owner of Ocean Art Pewter, made the first Comfort Heart (1996) and she continues to fill every order we give her. *May, I appreciate you so much.*

May asked her sister, Linda Power, also a cancer survivor, to work with me on the Comfort Heart Initiative, and over the next several years we worked hard to increase the awareness of Comfort Hearts.

Our partner of choice, then and now, is The Canadian Cancer Society. Some wonderful things have happened during this partnership. This small pewter heart has touched many individuals and has raised over **one and one half million dollars** for cancer research and other related projects within CCS.

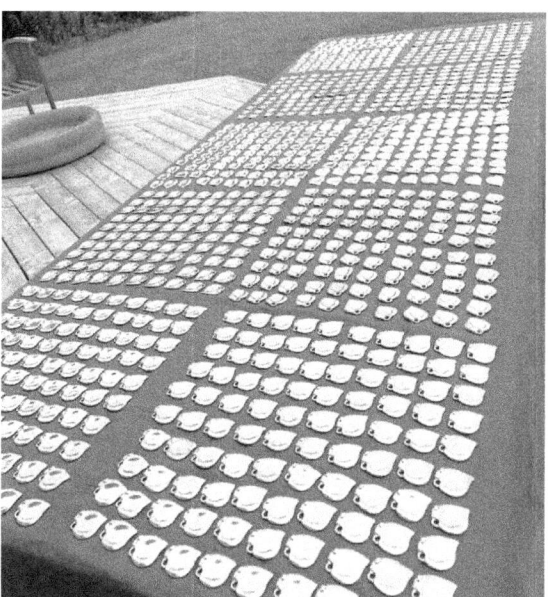

They say a picture is worth a thousand words. This picture is worth a thousand Comfort Hearts!

During the summer of 2021 May was filling an order for 500 hearts and, with one of her grandchildren helping, the total grew to 1000. Comfort Hearts were lined up on the ground just outside of May's home. Knowing May, I'm sure there was a 'teachable moment' or two during their discussions.

For the record, and I say this publicly as often as I can...

The Comfort Heart Initiative is not about me. It's about you.

Thank you for continuing to purchase hearts and thank you for sharing your stories with us. If you have a Comfort Heart, you are a member of my team that I proudly call the 'Holders of the Heart.'

This fundraiser began in 1996 and I received this note from Wendy Purcer dated October 5, 2023, proving the Comfort Heart Initiative is alive and well:

> Hi Carol Ann, I lost my 91year-old mother in June. I wear my Comfort Heart and press my thumb into the indentation to keep my mom close to me. Thank you for doing this so many years ago. I think of you and your mother often and I hope life is treating you well. Are the hearts still available?

They sure are, Wendy, and you can place your order by calling

1 888 939 3333.

Toni Hiltz, Executive Assistant with the Halifax office of The Canadian Cancer Society, wrote the following.

Hi Carol Ann,

As we catch a glimpse of a memory, it has the ability to make us laugh, cry, miss those who are no longer here...regardless of the emotion, memories bring comfort to our hearts. With just a single touch to the pewter Comfort Heart, you are transported to a memory that is totally yours.

Many have written or called us to share that your Comfort Heart brings warmth, and strength. For over a decade I have had the privilege to speak with people all over the world who wanted to purchase a Comfort Heart. Taking the time to listen to their stories, discovering what it means to them, brings a sense of strength and understanding and lets people know they are not alone.

It truly brings comfort to the heart.

Love,

Toni

Toni's Top Ten Uses for Comfort Hearts

1. Give it as a gift of comfort.
2. Put it on a bracelet or add a nice silk cord to turn it into a pendant.
3. Attach it to the sun visor of your vehicle.
4. Hang it from your key chain.
5. Have it as a personal touchstone.
6. With a red ribbon, use it as an ornament on your Christmas tree.
7. Give everyone in the family an engraved Comfort Heart.
8. Attach it to the zipper of your coat.
9. Clip it to a beloved pet's collar with name engraved on it.
10. Give a Comfort Heart as a token of thanks, for any occasion.

The Carol Ann Cole Comfort Heart Studentship Award

In 2011, Alyssa Patterson, a student at Mount Allison University in Sackville, New Brunswick, received the first Comfort Heart Studentship Award for breast cancer research.

The recipient of this award is able to continue his or her research in the lab during the summer months rather than having to secure a summer job to help raise the much-needed funds required to continue his or her studies.

Having met a number of our recipients, I can vouch for the fact that this award truly does allow a recipient to spend summers in the lab. It's much appreciated. I believe over the years I have received a personal thank you note from almost every recipient.

~

The Beatrice Hunter Cancer Research Institute (BHCRI) has undertaken rigorous peer reviews to ensure they are stewarding donor dollars for important research.

Additionally, BHCRI is involved with the Carol Ann Cole Comfort Heart

Studentship Award specifically for breast cancer research, as well as the new (2021) Carol Ann Cole Comfort Heart Graduate Award to be awarded to a Masters' or PhD student for cancer research (not specific to breast cancer).

~

Voula Pantelis is a friend of mine. She is also the General Manager of **Amoena***. Under the company name are the words "Supporting Confidence".*

That's what Amoena did for me following my second breast cancer battle. Voula opened a door or two for me and I have never forgotten her kindness. I asked Voula to update me on the world of Amoena.

2023-10-11
Dear Carol Ann,

Where would we be without women sharing their stories! You have made such an impact on so many, and helped others talk more openly about their journey with breast cancer.

Even after so many years as General Manager at Amoena Canada, I'm as amazed as I was on my first day what the effect of a breast form fitting has on a woman's healing.

Behind the fitting room curtain, your fitter sees your scars, sees any gaps you may have in your breast tissue and/or your chest wall and she sees YOU as unique, beautiful, present, and powerful.

If I was to describe Amoena in one word, I'd say it's transformative. We have been in business globally since 1975. Over 18 million breast forms later, we've taken the highest quality soft silicone forms to the next level in comfort, fit, and appearance.

Our latest breakthrough is using new technology to make garments that improve quality of life of women suffering from mild to moderate lymphedema in the thoracic area.

People often ask me what am I most proud of. I love the innovation. Amoena creations affirm that you are still you, still sensual, still beautiful. Amoena is about empowering women to own their story. It's healing.

I hope to see you soon...lunch in Toronto next time you're in town?
Voula

Part 4:

Mom and me

To be in your children's memories tomorrow, you have to be in their lives today

Anonymous

65: The world our grandchildren will inherit

What kind of a world are we leaving behind for those we love? It's a daunting question none of us can answer. That's of little help to our grandchildren.

Even if we have been, and continue to be, in their lives, we have to acknowledge that many of our grandchildren will grow up remembering their past life as pre-pandemic, followed by the ongoing pandemic. One day, we can only hope, they will live in a post-pandemic world. How do we make that a reality?

The year 2020 was a tough one that continued to hammer away at us through 2021 and well into 2023. Initially, I, like many of you, was frightened watching the number of COVID-19 patients entering the ICU departments of hospitals continue to rise in all provinces. What will our hospital system look like when our family has grown up?

Next up, we faced the Freedom Fighters, and, honestly, they frightened me. First they took over our country's capital and sat their 'big rigs' down for a month. Next, they seemed to splinter and pop up in smaller groups but large enough to make an impact in most communities. Many saw this as nothing more than a nuisance and to date, other than in Ottawa, I would agree. I found it difficult to read about protesters popping up telling us that not wearing a mask was their personal business. Protesters felt the country was trying to tell them to put a mask on rather than listen to their views, and they didn't like that. They wanted to be heard; however as they raised their voices, fewer people listened.

Early one Monday morning I listened to a Toronto doctor who was being interviewed during a local newscast. The doctor looked exhausted and angry as he told us about his weekend. He gave up his entire weekend with his family to sit with an ICU patient who was losing his battle with COVID. He didn't have anyone with him because they were not able to enter the hospital. His patient died. To wear a mask or not to wear a mask paled in comparison.

We certainly weren't prepared for what came next.

In February of 2022 we watched in horror as Russia invaded Ukraine, killing without consideration for the lives of women, children and babies, and men as well. It was utterly heartbreaking to watch the news. No one will ever forget the image of an injured mother-to-be who was in the throes of giving birth when the maternity hospital she was a patient in was bombed. Sadly, both mother and unborn baby boy died. Murdered, like so many others, at the hands of Russia.

As the war continued, it became clear that the Russians were not prepared for President Volodymyr Zelenskyy of Ukraine and his resolve. They underestimated the people's loyalty to home and country. Ukraine's soldiers and those who came from other countries to take up the battle... many who had yet to pick up a gun until they arrived... stood shoulder to shoulder to protect Ukraine.

As I watched this war continue to unfold, I found it difficult to give the freedom advocates any rental space in my head. My head was full of far more important and deadly stories.

There is only so much we as parents, grandparents and friends of the family can do to protect our younger families from all of this terrible news and, yes, some fake news, too. We do our best and we try to keep a close eye on our loved ones. There are days when the news is too much for some adults so imagine how difficult it must be for young children.

The 'good old days' are long gone as we carve new memories with our family. Some memories are created with a heavy heart, but in our ever-changing world we are learning as we go, and as long as we do the best we can, I believe our children and grandchildren will remember us that way...always, doing the best we can. So many things are beyond our reach.

I'm sure you have some thoughts. Please document here and share with your family. *Remember my offer to have you join me in the writing of this book?* This chapter would be a great place to document your thoughts regarding your own grandchildren and your hopes and dreams for them.

It takes time, energy, funds and a desire to be present in the lives of our children as we watch them grow and prepare to make their own mark in this world. It has never, leading up to and in the world we are part of in 2022-2024, been more important to make sure our connection to our families is stronger than ever before.

James Brian Scott, the boy, thank you. You have always remained present in my life and I'm so grateful. I appreciate you, my son.

Our children, grandchildren and others will not inherit our world; they will walk boldly into their own world.

Your thoughts:

66: Daughters and granddaughters

Let's teach the young women in our family to be....

Bold

Brave

Strong

Silly

Confident

Caring

Inclusive

Independent

Intelligent

Fierce

Funny

Teach your daughter to be a beautiful person,

Not just a pretty girl.

67: Mary Rose d'Entremont

My thoughts, as I write the final section of this book, are of my mother. I continue to learn from her every day. While she would definitely not be a fan of the Internet, I believe mom could relate to the quote below (I found it on the Internet!):

Be the woman
who fixes another woman's crown
without telling the world
it was crooked.

My mother was that woman.

My mother's parents, Evangeline and Marc d'Entremont, welcomed twelve children into the world. From the eldest to the baby of the family, they were Desire, Therese, Alphonse, Elise, Pauline, Marie Rose, Antionette, Emelina, Celine (died at birth), Roger (died at sixteen months), Denis and Andre.

They were all born at home. The dining room was turned into a birthing room twelve times!

I left home in June of 1964 for the bright lights of North Bay, Ontario. Initially I lived with my Aunt Edith and Uncle Ken plus their three sons, Chuck, Brian and Gary.

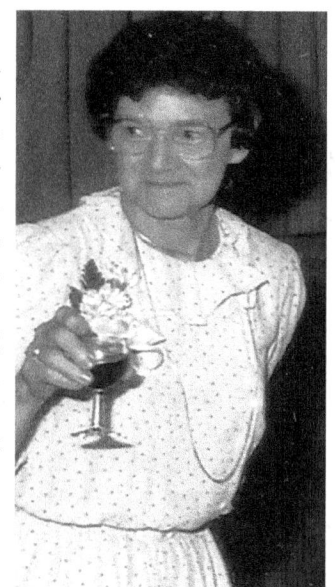

Aunt Edith was incredibly kind to me. She was a businesswoman in North Bay, holding down three jobs at any given time. She wanted to introduce me to the business world and she did exactly that.

Mom had saved $60 over a twelve-month period and she gave it to me as I was boarding the train in Halifax to move away from home, only a few days after my high school graduation.

Mom didn't use the same words, but she certainly prepared me to focus on always taking one step at a time and not giving up.

Many of my close friends and former MRHS classmates had left their hometowns and were working and living in Halifax. I knew this, but it still left me feeling alone when I arrived home one year later on my first vacation from the 'working world.' I no longer felt I was part of the 'in-crowd.' I didn't see it coming and it stung.

Since my friends were busy with the lives they had created for themselves, I hung out with mom. She treated me like an adult and I loved the new feelings I experienced of mother and daughter...sharing dreams. "It might be too late for my dreams to come true, Carol Ann, but your life is just beginning."

In that moment, standing with mom at the kitchen sink I realized, perhaps for the first time, how intelligent my mother was.

I realized, too, that mom had something on her mind, and if it was on her mind I wanted it on mine as well. I heard myself saying I was home for two weeks to help *her*.

I nudged mom...we were at the sink, shoulder to shoulder. "Mom, if you're finding it this difficult to share with me, I assume it's about dad... so spill."

Dad had gotten himself into a heap of trouble moneywise. In the eighteen years I lived at home I had never, *not once*, heard mom speak negatively about dad. And now she was heartbroken *and* blindsided to learn a mortgage had been taken out on our little Wilmot home. A mortgage that had been 'paid in full' some years ago. Someone had forged mom's signature. Dad's signature was his, for sure. No payments were being made.

I can't imagine how mom felt when she learned all of this. She had signed nothing. *Nothing.*

Having worked for a bank for an entire year, I felt certain I could march on down to Middleton and demand to see the bank manager. After all, I was a typist in the Bank of Nova Scotia in North Bay, so how much of a leap could it be for me to go head to head with the bank manager whom my dad spoke of as if they were best friends?

I acted without giving it a second thought. I took my teenage self and marched to Middleton, where I demanded to see the bank manager.

Looking around, I could see the manager in his office. I didn't wait for an invitation. I walked into his office with an attitude and a resolve to help my mother keep our home.

"Well now, you're one of Perry's girls, I believe. Lois, is it? Please take a seat and tell me what I can do for you. Can I assume you need a bit of money, Lois? My goodness, your father speaks so highly of you. Please sit."

"I'm good standing and, no, I am not Lois. I'm the second daughter, Carol Ann. Do you know I work in a bank? Believe me, I understand how mortgages are drawn up." That was a lie but he didn't know that.

I ranted and I raved about how I knew mom's signature on that mortgage had been forged and I wanted Mom to be given our house back. "And I want this mess cleaned up today. Today! I'm not leaving until you make this right. My mother is *not* moving out of her Wilmot home."

At that point in my rant the tide turned. I could feel it. Things did not go well...for me.

I was about to be kicked out of the bank, but not before being insulted. "Young lady, you have no idea what you are talking about. You're smart but you are no banker. Perry is right: you are a handful. He told me that a number of times. Get out of my bank. I'll even walk you to the curb."

I knew the manager would call my father the second I was out of the bank so I hurried home as fast as I could with my head down as I ran past the garage where dad worked.

Mom and I were in the living room and I was trying to remember every word the manager had said. "Mom, I knew he *would not* help us when he said if dad walked into his bank *right now* and asked for one thousand dollars he would loan it to him with no concern about dad's ability to make the payments in full and on time."

I wasn't sure if my mother was frightened for me or angry with me.

"Mom, I'm sorry. I will go to confession on Sunday...the last word I got to say was, 'bullshit' and *then* I left. Well, got kicked out is more accurate."

My mother was worried about how dad would react. "My land, Carol Ann, I wish you would have told me that's where you were going when you asked if you could go to Middleton. I would have found a way to stop you. I think you should be in your room when your father gets home for lunch. Let me talk to him first. You know 'that man'"—that's what she called the bank manager—"will have called your father and likely made things worse for all of us. I *hate* that man."

I don't think I had ever heard mom say that she hated anyone until that moment.

We didn't hear dad walk in. He came directly at us. It would be the last time my father would ever smack me upside the head.

My heart broke...for my mother and my two younger sisters. They would lose the only home they had ever known.

I was a teenager. There is an arrogance that sometimes comes with being a teenager, and while in the moment, I did not think I was being ar-rogant in any way I also did not do my homework. A bank typist of one year in another province is not an even match for a seasoned and well re-spected bank manager.

Lesson Learned? 'Once again, life is not fair.' Certainly, life was not fair to my mother.

Your thoughts:

68: A treasure trove

On January 23, 2020 the first identified case of COVID-19 in Canada during the pandemic was admitted to Sunnybrook Health Sciences Centre in Toronto. On March 17, the government of Ontario declared a state of emergency. This was followed by Toronto mayor John Tory declaring a local state of emergency on March 23.

I needed a new project! Ideally a project that involved writing, because I knew I could get lost in my writing and this would keep my mind occupied for some time.

This was my mom's cookbook.

I explored, with some excitement, the idea that mom's cookbook might, just might, contain more than cookbook stuff. I took my time and looked through the cookbook closely, beginning with the inside front cover.

I wanted to be certain that I hadn't overlooked anything and I couldn't do that if I began at the centre of mom's 'cookbook journal', as we called it. This cookbook opened at the centre quite naturally because that's where all the pasting of her favourite recipes ended up. The last half of her journal had fooled me for many years. I just assumed there

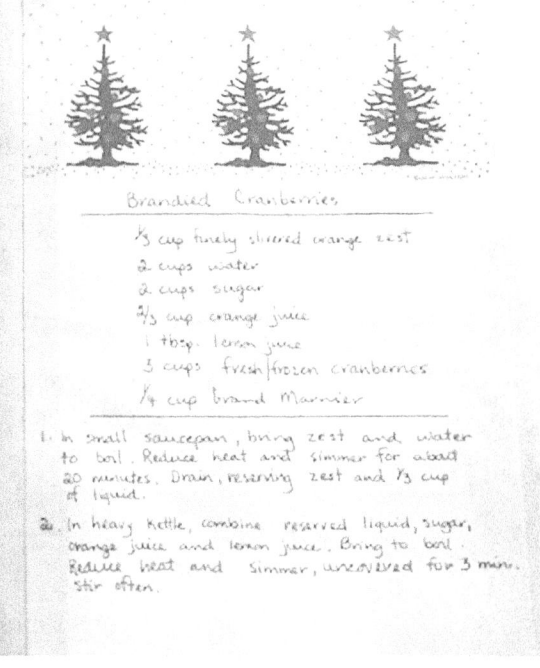

was nothing in the first half.

And what did I find between the pages in the first half of Mom's journal? *A treasure trove.* I could feel my mother's energy. I learned so much more about mom as I read her words. It was as if she was sitting right beside me.

As it turns out, mom liked to keep her 'good stuff' all in one place. She passed that love on to me. I am proud to share a small part of my mother's good stuff, much of it written in her own hand. There was no 'cut and paste' during Mom's era.

As you read the following you will see mom's writing was always about her family...her girls.

Love, like the ocean, is vast and forever.
Sorrow is but a shadow that moves over the sea.

~

Count your nights by stars, not shadows.
Count your life by smiles, not tears.
With joy on every birthday...
Count your age by friends...not years.

~

A mother is someone who sends her children into the future,
Wishing them love and laughter.
Handing them a pack to carry as they go,
Filled with hope, dreams and happy memories.

~

Time is a mystery. It comes and it goes.
Although you can't see it, in the mirror, it shows.
I believe in the sun even when it doesn't shine.
I believe in love even when it's not shown.
I believe in God,
Even when he doesn't speak.

~

Perhaps nobody becomes more competent
in hitting a moving target
Than a mother spoon-feeding her baby.

I have wonderful memories of my mother with her friends, 'the five sisters', living in Halifax. Mom and I were on a plane that would take us from Toronto home to Halifax. I had a business meeting with Aliant (circa 1990) and I invited mom to make the trip with me. She was thrilled. We would stay in the city for a few days following my meetings.

This was before we battled cancer (1992) and before we would learn just how hard mom would have to fight to carve out less than a year following her surgery and treatments.

We flew home, checked into our hotel, had a bite to eat, and then we walked along the beautiful Halifax boardwalk. We were both so drawn to this area of the city. For us, there was nothing like Halifax harbour and sitting on one of the many chairs positioned from one end of the boardwalk to the other.

The weather was perfect, the boardwalk was ripe with locals, it was a wonderful evening.

Suddenly mom smiled, saying, rather loudly I thought, "Oh my land!"

She spread her arms wide, seemingly in recognition of five women walking towards us. They were totally unfamiliar to me.

Their smiles turned to laughter as they lined up to hug 'Mary', as each of the sisters said in turn. It was easy to see that they were sisters.

Mom made a very fast introduction followed by, "Carol Ann, why don't you *go on back* to the hotel. My friends will make sure I get back to you safely."

Just like that I was dismissed. *And I loved it!*

Off they went, leaving me in their dust! Melva, Betty, Rosalie, Audrey and Natalie knew mom from her working days at the old Halifax Infirmary. Rosalie shares a birthday with mom and, combining birthdays with Christmas, they celebrated together every year in December.

Mom had trained the youngest of the sisters, Natalie, to work in the Sterilization Department of the Infirmary. Among mom's journals was a black 'scribbler', as we called them back-in-the-day, and inside mom had carefully written all the instructions, not only for the sterilization but also the placement of instruments on trays for different surgeries. This job had been a promotion for mom and she was grateful, as she was for everything in her life. Perhaps a few exceptions, but we all have those.

Audrey, who now lives in Ontario to be closer to her own large family, comes home pretty much every summer for two months to be with her sisters in the home where they grew up. The sisters own their home and are very proud of that accomplishment...and they should be. They are kept busy with many projects, one at a time: preparing for a new deck, a new lawn, a new bathroom, a new kitchen...you get the picture!

Large projects do not frighten these ladies. They hire a man they have trusted for years. No job was too big to take on.

On a cold winter's day, March 9, 2022, I wrapped mom's black scribbler in tissue, found a nice bag to put it in, tied it with a red ribbon, and set out to meet the sisters for lunch. I surprised them when I presented my mom's gift after so many years.

It was an emotional moment, recalling their memories of their friend, Mary. They recognized her writing immediately. "This is actually in Mary's writing!"

By the time everyone had a look at mom's signature we were all in tears.

It is a pleasure staying in touch with such good friends of my mother. Now I call them friends of mine, and I know mom would be so happy to see us all together, walking the boardwalk just as she did with her good friends, the sisters, so many years ago.

We could learn so much from observing how these ladies live their lives. I asked if I could help them write their own story. They felt this mention about them with 'Mary' was enough!

69: Mom's love of reading

Mom loved to read and she loved to journal. Not counting her twenty-two books about the Royal Family, mom noted in her diary that in total she had read over two hundred books! She gave each book a rating: excellent, very good, good, special, funny, emotional and, the lowest of all, stupid!

Mom, like many of her friends, loved her family but wasn't afraid to say she was happy on her own, too. She often spent her alone time reading.

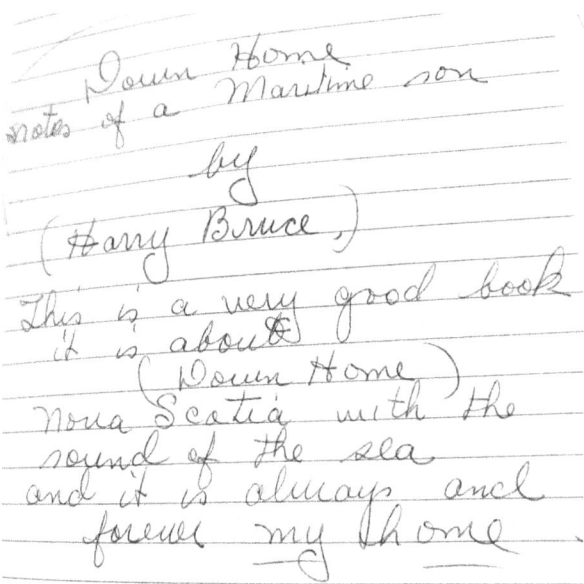

Down Home by Harry Bruce was one of mom's favourite books. 'The sound of the sea, and forever my home.'

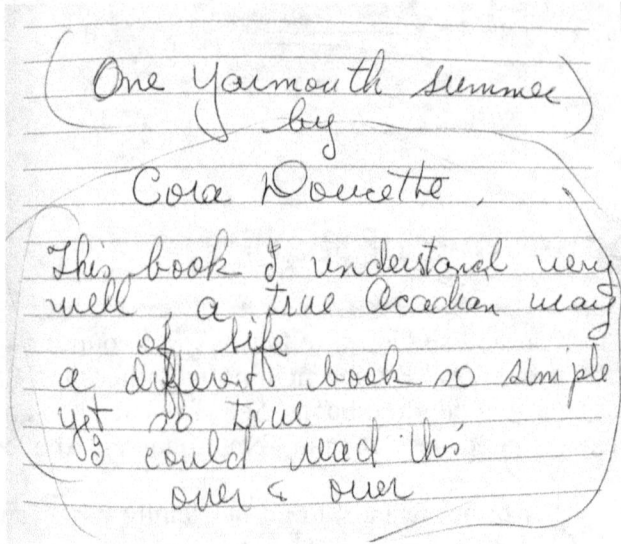

(One Yarmouth summer)
by
Cora Doucette.

This book I understand very well, a true Acadian way of life a different book so simple yet so true I could read this over & over

Cora Doucette wrote *One Yarmouth Summer*. Being of Acadian blood herself Mom appreciated the true Acadian way of life.

Your thoughts:

70: Oh, what a party!

My sisters and I planned a 75th birthday party for mom. Lois came home from Grande Prairie, Lorraine from Calgary and Connie from Honolulu.

Mom's sister, Anne, and brother, Andy, came into Toronto from Hamilton, along with their spouses, Paul and Nora. Cousins, friends and neighbours joined the party. Mom was thrilled and so happy.

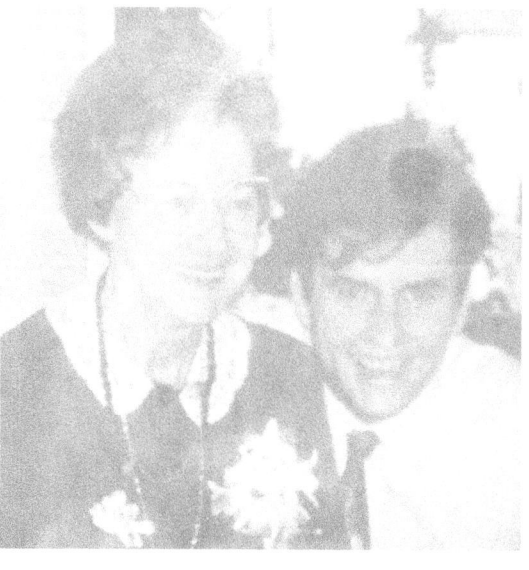

James knelt by mom's side off and on for hours. He was in charge of monitoring the enter-phone in the lobby to let our guests in. Mom was very proud of her grandson. To watch my son and my mother sharing so many smiles filled my heart with gratitude.

At one point James offered the chance for everyone to smile. "Grandmother, I don't remember your brother or your sister's names. I have no idea who most of these people are. We better stop letting everyone in, so I'm officially off duty. I've been letting *everyone* in, by the way. That stops now! All good with you?"

As 'Mary's girls', the four of us were thrilled as each of mom's guests arrived. Mom didn't know who was coming, so literally each person was a surprise. The party was a great success.

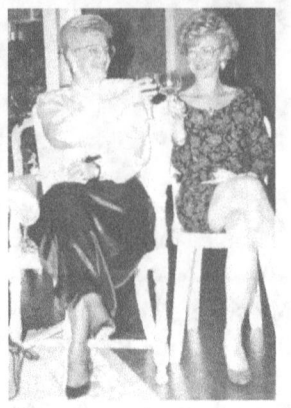

I snapped this picture of Lois and Connie 'toasting' mom during the celebration. I was so happy that my three sisters were able to come to Toronto from so far away.

Mom wrote, from her heart, in her diary about her birthday party when she returned home that very evening. Lorraine got in the limo with mom and went home with her for a few days. My sisters and I still talk about how glowing our mother was that evening. You can see from her journal entry just how much the party meant to her.

Sat, Nov 17 1990
my family had a party for my 75th birthday with my family and many friends it was a special evening for me I can not put in words how I felt that night. I'll always have in my heart happy memories of that night.

Thank you
Carol Ann
Lois,
Lorraine
Connie
Tom

71: We didn't know

Fast forward to one year later. November, 1991.

(1991)

Nov 17° to Nov 24ᵗʰ.
a week in N.B. with
my sister, for us its
always a special time
to be together, just to
talk and share past
memories of long ago.
Had a good flight home
now to unpack, and get
to bed, I'm tired, have so
much mail here including
Christmas cards and letters
from everybody.

(a great week for me)

Mom visited with her sister, Pauline, in New Brunswick and her diary entry offers a hint of the wonderful time they had together. Mom would never speak of favouring one sibling over another, but I do believe she and Aunt Pauline were true best friends. Mom loved her sister's family, too!

Connie, and her late husband, John Dea, visited Aunt Pauline each time they vacationed in Nova Scotia. Like mom, Connie had a lovely relationship with Aunt Pauline.

Mom shared her gratitude with her niece, Anna, and Ed Taylor, as they came with us to Saint Michel's Cathedral in downtown Toronto for midnight mass. Mom loved midnight mass and she loved Anna. When we were young, and when we could be sure of a safe ride to and from our church, Mom and her girls went to midnight mass at Saint Monica's Catholic Church in Middleton... whether we wanted to or not.

December 25th, 1991 James and I took mom to the Old Mill restaurant for their beautiful Christmas buffet.

Mom was always happy to spend Christmas with James and me.

In retrospect, it's as if she had already made the hard decision and knew exactly what she would face in the New Year. With the decision made, mom was able to compartmentalize this and enjoy Christmas Day! She was incredibly strong that way.

> Dec 24.
> (Christmas Eve.)
> So many memories for me
> now there just shadows
> To-night is a time to remember
> all the good, this is such
> a special night,
> Christmas Eve Mass.
> is something so special
> for me,
> Carol Ann, Anna, Edward
> and I we went to
> St. Michael's Basilica
> it was a lovely service
> for me Christmas Eve
> Mass is a special
> night always has been.
>
> after we came home
> we opened all the gifts
> that's the first time ever for
> me, I we always opened
> the gifts on Christmas morning

72: Mary's girls surround her

Mom's journal entry dated January 1st, 1992 speaks volumes. All of our lives changed before the month was over.

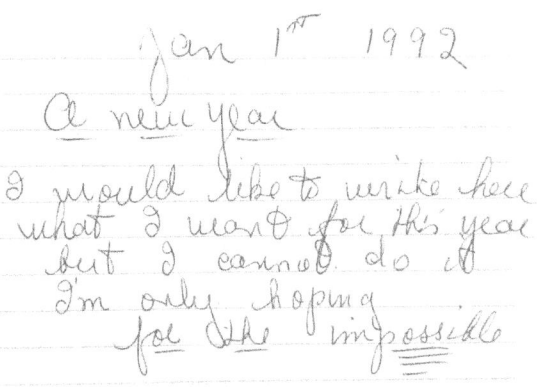

Jan 1st 1992

A new year

I would like to write here what I want for this year but I cannot do it I'm only hoping for the impossible

Mom was at the point where she was going to have to book an appointment with her doctor. In her heart of hearts, she knew what she would be facing simply by making the appointment.

A mere few days later both mom and I would be facing our own battles with breast cancer. *Dark days.*

Mom could pull herself up and win her fight of the day, and she did that for eleven months. As you will see in a few entries below, following surgery and then being told she had metastatic breast cancer, her resolve remained strong. There were certain things she wanted to do. She had plans to live to the very end...then she would think about her own death.

My granddaughter, Lexi, has my mother's 'I can do it.' attitude and I love that so much.

When mom gave me her journals, we went through them one by one and page by page to ensure she was happy with me having so much knowledge about her thoughts and dreams. She did ask me to rip out a number of pages, and we threw out some entire journals. We destroyed over half her diaries at her request and she may have destroyed more than a few of her journals even before she moved in with me.

"You girls don't need to read about my dreams that turned into mere shadows of all that I had hoped for. All my hopes and dreams are gone, and that's that." So like mom to tell you what she was feeling and, sure enough, that was that.

Mom's comment, "My memories became merely shadows," is sprinkled through a number of her journals. If you knew mom at all, you would agree that this is the most negative thing that would escape her lips.

> in the hospital 6 days,
> from this day on whatever
> will happen I don't know,
> only God knows,
> but I can live with it
> sunshine or darkness
> I will make the best of it
> I can do it.

Mom wasn't sure about this page in her diary. In the end, we ripped the top half of the page off because it was more personal than she wanted to share.

Mom always smiled whenever I mentioned that I would like to one day publish her written words. "My land, Carol Ann, no one cares what I've written down on paper. I worry you will be disappointed, so make sure I'm dead when you publish this stuff."

Mom smiled as she made this last statement and I tried to convince her that what she had to say was important and others could learn from her. She wasn't convinced, but I had her support to go ahead...one day in the future and long after the year 1992.

The night before my own breast cancer surgery, and only a couple weeks after her diagnosis and surgery, mom wrote the following in her journal. When I read these words for the first time I was incredibly touched. It certainly made me cry.

Her words, with not a mention of what she had already been through in the same month, were so like my mother. Her first thoughts were always of her four girls. On this particular day, January 27, 1992, I had top billing...at least for a week or two.

In February, 1992, Lois came home for a month and she brought her portable sewing machine along! I was so impressed, honestly. Mom loved having her eldest daughter with her.

First thing on their list was to actually make a list to ensure all the projects mom had for Lois would be completed. Their list was so long it made me dizzy. Lots of sewing and spring-cleaning (in February) Mom's entire little apartment. Baking. Cooking. Laundry, and that meant both starching and ironing everything...and I do mean everything.

The month flew by and on March 28th it was time to pick Lois up at Mom's and get her settled in at the Toronto airport. Mom's journal entry the day Lois flew home to Grande Prairie spoke volumes. She was sad to see her leave and Lois was worried about leaving mom not knowing what would come next. They had had so much fun together and Lois did so many things for her.

As Lois and I were carrying her sewing machine and her luggage to the elevator, mom walked with us. They hugged and hugged again. Finally, I had a question for them.

"Hello, ladies, do you know what day it is today?"

Lois was quick to say, "Am I going to the airport on the wrong day?"

And my own mother said, "Carol Ann, of course we know what day it is. What are you talking about?"

"Today is my birthday!"

They looked at each other as if in shock. I had certainly been successful in lightening the mood!

I continued to speak about this, all in good humour, whenever mom and I were having a bad day. We had more than a few of those, but with mom's resolve, she would manage to pull us both out of our slump. I did what I could.

In later years when I read mom's diary for March 28, 1992 there it was. The day her first-born flew home and my birthday.

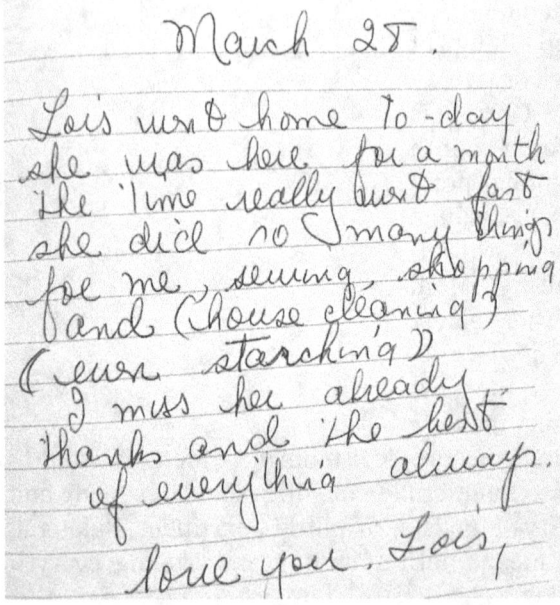

We celebrated Mother's Day, where else but at The Old Mill. Mom couldn't eat much, and for the most part did not feel well. Metastatic breast cancer can do that to you. But never a negative word about it from my strong Acadian mother.

A wonderful memory was made on this particular Mother's Day. Mom did not believe in 'playing the cancer card' and she had made that very clear. "Do *not* mention cancer when we're out in public."

When James and I picked Mom up she looked beautiful, with a bit of make-up on, a beautiful dress, lovely scarf and her signature smile shining brightly. This was to be a cancer-free day. No mention of cancer and no saying, "Are you okay? Do you need help?" Again, got it, mom.

We parked the car and walked to the restaurant, only to find a line up a mile long. I knew mom could not stand in line and I also knew I could say nothing about it. I had promised.

After about twenty seconds of standing in line my tiny mother leaned in and said, "Carol Ann, I want you to go to the front of this line right now and tell somebody I have cancer. You'll have to butt in and get ahead of everyone and you know how I hate seeing people do that. I need to sit down. I've got cancer and I feel unwell. Can you make that happen?"

Done! (And I played our cancer card times-two until the server and I were both crying.) In mere minutes we had the best seat in the house with two glasses of bubbly on our table before we even sat down. My mother did not drink, so, before eating anything, I had two glasses of bubbly. James' drink of choice was a Coke. A very special Mother's Day happened that day.

From Mother's Day until mom's last day later that same year, I would threaten to approach someone in any lineup we faced, and play the cancer card. We laughed every time.

Next up was a special trip for mom and one she had asked us to make happen for her.

Lorraine joined mom and me as we headed to Niagara on the Lake for a few days of rest. We walked around a bit and ate according to how mom was feeling. Lorraine convinced us we needed a well-balanced meal, so that's what we had...for every meal!

During our stay, Lorraine and I shared a room with a door into mom's room. Each night, when mom was tucked in, we talked about what the next few months would look like for mom and how I might help her...and help myself as well. Lorraine taught me so much during that trip.

Lorraine and Tom had made it clear that I could call them anytime and as often as required. If I needed them to come to Toronto, they would book the first flight out of Calgary, no questions asked. During those times when I panicked and said I needed their help, it was never suggested that their trip was not necessary after all.

Watching mom battle cancer as I was attempting to recover from my own was draining even more than I wanted to admit. Lorraine and Tom understood.

Mom had hopes to travel to Ottawa 'one more time.' She loved everything about our country's beautiful capital. This trip was definitely on mom's list of things to do. Today, we would call it a bucket list.

The trip meant so much to mom and she smiled through her pain the entire time we were there. Cancer was trying to win but mom had more living to do. Her humour was evident. "We drove to the Capitol, not to see Brian [Mulroney], but to visit the beautiful buildings here."

Our final trip was to Halifax to attend the Military Tattoo. Mom loved going to the Tattoo and you could see the excitement in her eyes and in every step she took on our 'Tattoo day.'

Connie flew home from Honolulu and Mom was so happy to have her in Halifax with us.

Sadly, our beautiful mother was feeling quite ill and had to fight very hard to enjoy the city she loved so much. Early in the Tattoo performances mom asked us to take her back to our hotel. We knew how terrible she was feeling simply because she had asked to leave. This was a first.

We got her into a cab and asked if she would rather we take her to emergency. Her response was so like mom. "Well, I hate to ruin your evening but if you girls don't mind, I better see a doctor."

The emergency room doctor couldn't believe mom had flown to Halifax 'in the state she is in.' Connie and I were insulted when he asked if either of us had any idea how sick our mother was. We let it go without a comment and kept our total focus on mom.

Following a full day in the city with mom and Connie after the Tattoo and our experience in taking mom to emergency, I had to cut my trip short and fly back to Toronto. I would soon return to work and wanted to be 'ready.' I had been off work for almost six months, giving myself time to heal. This also gave my sisters and me the time to fulfill many of mom's hopes and dreams.

Connie stayed in Halifax with mom for the week. They had a wonderful time together and made their own memories.

Once back in Toronto, Mom wrote, "I don't feel well at all. What is coming? But this trip was something I'll remember always...because we were together."

73: A final diary entry

The last entry in mom's diary is dated September 5, 1992 and it will break your heart. James came home to be with us as we moved mom from her apartment in Scarborough, Ontario to my condo. I looked after the movers working in mom's apartment and James looked after his grandmother.

> Sept 5.
>
> To-day I moved in with Carol Ann I have a lovely (small apartment) and with all my own things it will feel like home as I had all things are for me I'll be happy and safe here, I know the girls will always look after me
> Well the end,

James made sure he took as much time with her as possible so that I had time to get her new apartment in order. By the time they arrived in downtown Toronto, the master bedroom had been turned into mom's private suite, including a large bathroom. Her living-room furniture fit easily. As a surprise, we brought her 'good' dishes that she had suggested we give away.

Mom sat at the table for each meal and she always had the table looking lovely. A lady to the end…always using her 'good' dishes.

The final sentence in Mom's diary (above) says it all. "I'll be happy and safe here. I know the girls will look after me until the end."

Even in death, my mother is a tough act to follow.

Your thoughts:

74: Cole's Corner

What I hope you are able to feel while reading some of mom's journal entries is that she *never gave up*. She was positive to the end, with very few blips along the way. Mom knew how her story would end. Her 'I can do it' attitude served her well. I am so grateful that she shared that attitude with me.

Good dishes

A couple of months after moving in with me, mom gathered up a bit of energy so we could have a short conversation.

"Carol Ann, I never thanked you for the surprise when you brought my good dishes from my apartment to your home. That made me happy. I felt so good when both you and James reminded me that this is our home now not your home. It really does feel like *our* home, Carol Ann. Thank you for that, too."

Giving thanks to the end...that was so like our mother.

The decision to bring the dishes was an easy one. They were her 'good dishes' and she used them at every meal. She worried there wouldn't be room for her dishes in my kitchen.

First I said, "It's *our* kitchen now." Putting an arm around mom, I added, "Don't confuse me with your three other daughters. I'm the one who doesn't 'do kitchen,' remember?"

Just before 6 am most days I locked my condo door and went to a local fitness centre only minutes away. When I returned an hour or so later Mom would be up, bed made, dressed and sitting at the table with her good dishes laid out as she enjoyed her breakfast. I carry that image in my mind and my heart always.

Glitz and glam

This picture was taken mid 1992. Brian (Bastedo) and I were going to a Bell function and this was my first 'appearance' post breast cancer surgery and twenty-eight radiation treatments.

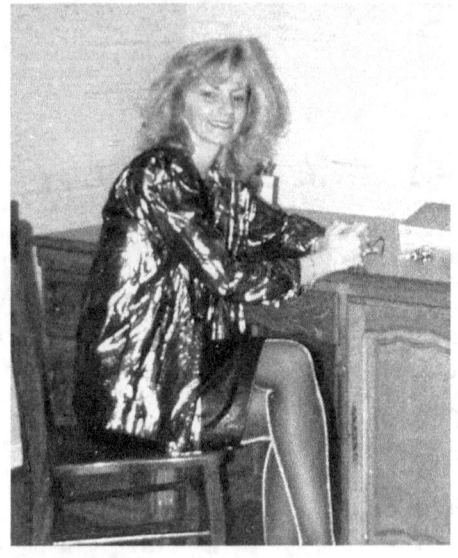

During the days leading up to the gala I had admitted to my mother that I was lacking a bit of confidence and was feeling anxious. I mentioned my pre-radiation 'tattoos' still being visible high on my breast bone and into my underarm area.

Mom's immediate response was, "My land, Carol Ann, you and I can go shopping for something glittery and bright that has long sleeves and can be buttoned up to your neck if you want. And, by the way, I don't think that is necessary. After all, they're not real tattoos. *Are they?* If anyone spots one of your tattoos I believe you should wear them proudly."

I thanked mom for the gentle slap upside the head.

It was mom who found this black-and-silver glittery blouse with a matching camisole. I bought it, buttoned it up, tucked it into my little black ruffled short skirt, added my glam-hosery and my Bruno Magli heels and I was ready to go.

The only reason I mention the brand of shoes here is that the heel was not the killer-high-heeled shoe that made up part of my personal dress code. I had given myself this gift of a pair of 'Made in Italy' shoes. I wanted to be able to dance all night and I hadn't worn heels in six months. We danced and we danced and we danced. When Brian and I were not on the dance floor, many of my peers and my own team dropped by our table to say hi and to welcome me back. And, just like that, my confidence was back.

I'm a firm believer that when you treat yourself, you should treat someone you love as well. It doesn't have to be Italian leather shoes; it can be an ice-cream cone on a sunny day. For now, I'm still looking for the right person to gift my 'special' shoes to.

Don't second-guess your decisions

It would be easy to say, 'Make the right decision in the first place,' but we all know that doesn't always happen. If you make a bad decision, make sure you learn something from the experience. And don't make the same decision again.

This story dates back to my radiation treatments in 1992. I would later learn that those treatments had, in error, damaged my left lung and caused me to have a bitter cough that often turned into pneumonia when left untreated.

I had an appointment to meet with my radiation oncologist after I finished twenty-eight treatments. His first questions were, "Tell me about that cough. When did it start? How long has it been as bad as it seems to be today? Are you able to sleep?"

He then proceeded to share that this would undoubtedly be radiation pneumanitas and I might have it for life. He did offer to put me on steroids but emphasized that that would mean I would be on a steroid for life. I decided to learn to live with it.

I asked how this could happen. How could I have life-long lung damage following radiation treatments to my breast after the removal of a small cancerous tumour? My breast seemed to be a long way from my lung, yes?

The doctor's reply was swift. "It is possible to damage the lung of a skinny and flat-chested woman who presents with breast cancer and requires radiation."

I suggested, in future, he might say, "Slim and small breasted," so as not to further insult the patient.

His reply was brief: "Point taken."

End of discussion.

I made a conscious decision to move forward in my recovery. I was forty-five years old and had lots of living to do.

First I wanted to regain my health so I could return to work. Second, my sisters and I knew early in 1992 that mom's recovery would be nothing like mine. My cancer was stage one; mom's was not. I wanted to be present for my mother.

Fast forward to today, and I try very hard to not second-guess my decision in 1992. I now have a chronic lung disease, in part because of the radiation damage to my left lung, in error!

At every opportunity I encourage other breast cancer patients to ask why every single tattoo placed on their breast prior to radiation treatments is in that exact spot and is there any chance it might slip a bit and harm a major organ...like their lungs for example.

I did attempt to contact my former radiation oncologist to try to understand more about the placement of tattoos. He was gone from my hospital. I believe he went into private practice and then back with one of the big hospitals on University Avenue, and now I understand he is in the USA.

Mom had five radiation treatments and later one more in an attempt to ease the pain she was experiencing at the base of her spine. Each day, as her name was called and I watched mom disappear into a room where, once the radiation beams were matched with the tattoos on her tiny battered body, she would take another radiation hit, I marvelled at her resolve to accept all of this.

Mom, if I could speak with you today I would tell you that while I do think back to our cancer experience together I reflect on only the good moments. You were able to compartmentalize cancer, and for the eleven months you lived following those dark days in January of 1992, you were *living*, not dying. And you never complained, not one single time.

Lois inherited that from you, mom and to this day, even when I beg her to complain about one little thing...she does not do it. She simply doesn't complain.

My dear mother, Mary Rose d'Entremont...

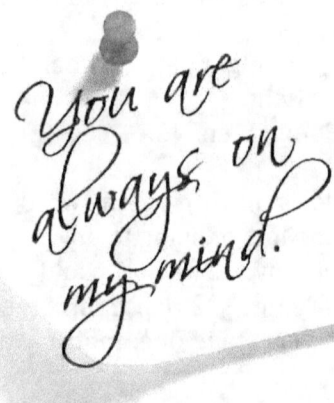

Back-from-away

Anywhere in Nova Scotia I would be called a 'back-from-away', meaning I once lived here and now I'm back. The 'come-from-away' folks have moved here but have not previously lived in our beautiful province.

In the summer of 2021 I purchased a tiny condo in downtown Halifax. I could not be happier. I have written and rewritten this entire book sitting in my mother's rocking chair and looking at Halifax Harbour. I hope my happiness is reflected in my writing.

Allow your 'comfort zone' to grow and develop

As we age, we can become more hesitant to try something new. It becomes more difficult to step out of our comfort zone. If we could only retain that childhood feeling that we could do anything, should do everything and would do it all.

I have lots of pictures of my grandchildren, and this one of Lexi is one of my favourites. As she inspected the inside of the dishwasher it was clear that she was in her comfort zone.

As I approached Lexi, I could imagine her young mind thinking, "I can't be in trouble already. I just got up. Go ahead...take my picture."

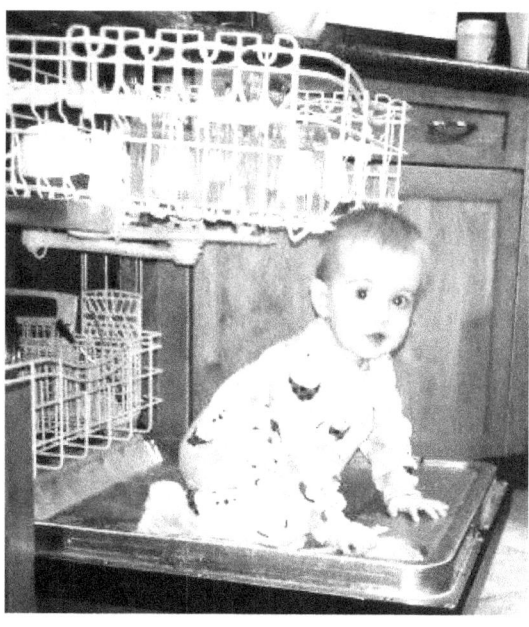

As I end this very long letter to each of you, please remember to be kind. Help your family and your friends. Help a stranger. Listen...everything else will follow.

I encourage you to live your personal 'Dash' wisely. If you falter today there is always tomorrow and tomorrow comes with a clean slate. Remember that.

Make that phone call you have been thinking you should make. Do it now. Don't wait until you 'have time', because, as we all know, this rarely happens.

Visit the family member who has been on your mind. I find that COVID, in spite of all of its ugliness, also brought us together like never before. My sisters and I began meeting monthly via Zoom. We love 'seeing' each other on a regular basis.

Personally, I find that I now reach out to more of my fellow Coles, and some for the first time, to be honest. That's on me.

I hope you have enjoyed this book, and I hope you take advantage of my offer to share the blank pages with you. Jot down memories that you hope others will draw on when you are no longer around. I have left room for you on many pages.

Share funny lines and funny stories that your family will understand. They will smile knowingly and they may silently thank you for your note.

It's okay to be sad when you make your notes, too...that makes you real.

I have included some very personal experiences that I have not shared before. You might not want to be as personal with your notes, and that, too, is okay.

Finally...a reminder for everyone.

I hope you'll dance.

I danced growing up and certainly in high school at the "Teen Town" dances at our MRHS.

I danced with my husband. Graydon and I loved to dance, and in our early days together we danced often.

When James and I were first on our own, and remember we pretty much grew up together, we danced just because we wanted to. Sometimes we danced together. Sometimes we danced on our own, but always in view of each other, which brought smiles and laughs from both of us. Oh, how we danced.

Today my son, his wife Tracey, Jalen and Lexi are all great dancers.

And they dance often...example being the 'dance parties' Jalen and Lexi enjoyed almost every evening just after supper as they were growing up.

I loved those moments and I love the memories they have given me.

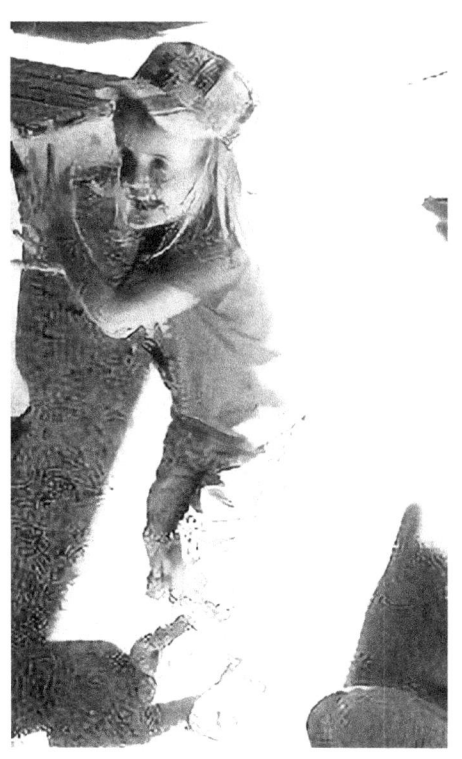

With love always, from the heart,

Carol Ann

PS at the risk of repeating myself, always remember...

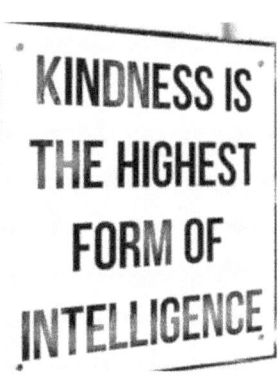

Your thoughts:

Acknowledgements

Thank you to my Wilmot friend, Phyllis Pedicelli, for painting the cover.

Moose House Publications is the perfect home for my books. Thank you to Brenda Thompson, my publisher, and to Andrew Wetmore, my editor, who keeps my mind sharp.

This is my first non fiction in over a decade. Thank you to all who have contributed to this book and to everyone I have contacted during the writing of it. Thank you to everyone I have contacted to seek permission to include all or part of your work here.

Thank you to all who have supported and enjoyed my non-fiction work in the past. I hope you will add this book to your library.

Learning to Slow Dance

About the author

Carol Ann Cole C. M. is a best-selling author, a professional speaker and the founder of the Comfort Heart Initiative in memory of her mother, Mary Rose d'Entremont, who is featured on many pages of this book.

Learning to Slow Dance with Footprints of Kindness is Carol Ann's fifth non-fiction book. She is also the author of five novels in The Paradise Series.

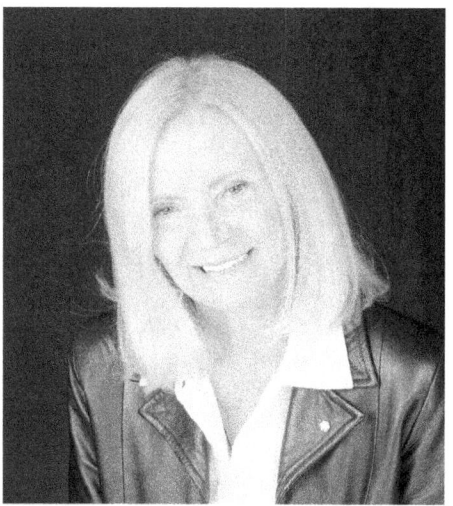

www.ingramcontent.com/pod-product-compliance
Lightning Source LLC
Chambersburg PA
CBHW061150120626
46546CB00005B/2003